SO-AWB-221

## Research Resources and Implications for Occupational Therapy

# OUTCOMES OF STROKE REHABILITATION

*Editors*
Patricia C. Ostrow, MA, OTR, FAOTA
Deborah Lieberman, MA, OTR/L
Susan C. Merrill, MA, OTR

*Quantitative Synthesis by*
Kenneth J. Ottenbacher, PhD, OTR, FAOTA

*Assistant Editors*
Kathy L. Kaplan, MS, OTR
Barbara E. Joe, MA

*Foreword by*
John W. Williamson, MD

The American Occupational Therapy Association, Inc.
Rockville, Maryland

RC
388.5
087
1985

LC

The American Occupational Therapy Association, Inc.
1383 Piccard Drive
Rockville, MD 20850

Copyright 1985 by the American Occupational Therapy Association, Inc.
All rights reserved. Published 1985
Printed in the United States of America

The following publishers have generously given permission to use adapted versions of copyrighted article abstracts appearing in their periodicals: Abstract nos. 1, 13--reprinted by permission of Lancet Publications; nos. 2-4, 6, 7, 9, 18, 27, 33, 39, 43, 46-48, 51, 53, 59, 61, 64, 67, 73, 75, 77, 78--reprinted by permission of the American Congress of Rehabilitation Medicine; no. 5--reprinted by permission of the International Rehabilitation Medicine Association; nos. 10, 28, 29, 30, 63--reprinted by permission of the British Medical Association; nos. 11, 19-21, 23, 25, 68, 72--reprinted by permission of the American Heart Association, Inc.; no. 14--reprinted by permission of the College of Physicians Update Publications, Ltd.; nos. 15, 31, 42--reprinted by permission of Bailliere Tindall; no. 16--reprinted by permission of Oxford University Press; no. 17--reprinted by permission of the Helen Dwight Reid Educational Foundation; nos. 22, 24--reprinted by permission of the Medical Society of the State of New York; nos. 26, 32--reprinted by permission of Paragon Press, Inc.; nos. 35, 69--reprinted by permission of W. B. Saunders Co.; no. 36--reprinted by permission of Almqvist and Wiksell International; no. 37--reprinted by permission of the North Carolina Occupational Therapy Association; nos. 38, 40, 58--reprinted by permission of the American Physical Therapy Association, Inc.; nos. 41, 54, 65--reprinted by permission of the Controller, Her Majesty's Stationery Office; nos. 45, 50--reprinted by permission of the Medical Journal of Australia; no. 49--reprinted by permission of the American Geriatrics Society; no. 52--reprinted by permission of the Minnesota State Medical Association; no. 56--reprinted by permission of the Haworth Press; no. 57--reprinted by permission of the American Academy of Family Physicians; no. 60--reprinted by permission of Excerpta Medica; no. 62--reprinted by permission of John Wright & Sons, Ltd.; no. 70--reprinted by permission of the Singapore Medical Association; no. 76--reprinted by permission of the Missouri State Medical Association.

**LIBRARY OF CONGRESS CATALOGING IN PUBLICATION DATA**

Main entry under title:

Outcomes of stroke rehabilitation.

   Bibliography: p.
   Includes index.
   1. Cerebrovascular disease--Patients--Rehabilitation--
Abstracts.   2. Occupational therapy--Abstracts.
I. Ostrow, Patricia Curran, 1930-   .   II. Lieberman,
Deborah.   III. Merrill, Susan Cook.   IV. American
Occupational Therapy Association.
RC388.5.O87   1985      616.8'1        85-20109
ISBN 0-910317-18-6

1-7-89

# CONTENTS

# FOREWORD

This book on outcomes of stroke rehabilitation has importance that far outweighs the meaningful information it provides to occupational therapists and other health professionals for improving the management of stroke patients. It offers a model that can be used by health organizations in the difficult task of making readily accessible the relevant and valid science information required for health care decisions. The evidence of recent studies strongly corroborates practitioners' experience with the problem of screening the burgeoning medical literature, only a small proportion of whose articles are both scientifically sound and relevant to practitioners for immediate decision making.

It is unreasonable to expect that individual health care professionals can successfully cope with this problem. It is reasonable and necessary, as this book demonstrates, that national organizations assume the responsibility of science information management for their members and constituents. The American Occupational Therapy Association (AOTA) has done so, allocating scarce internal resources to provide such a service to its members by means of the Efficacy Data Project. This pioneering effort will, in my opinion, prove to be a landmark development in leading the way for other health organizations to undertake similar projects.

What, in fact, does this book represent to justify the above assertions? It exemplifies a new type of publication variously termed information synthesis and validated review. What is unique about this type of publication is that it delineates, in sufficient detail, the methods applied to compile and validate its contents according to three critical criteria, namely, that the information reported be--

1. Representative of available scholarly work on the topic studied, though not necessarily exhaustive;
2. Valid scientifically in terms of its quantitative or heuristic value;
3. Replicable in terms of the documentation provided.

With reference to the first criterion (representativeness), building a data or information base that might be judged "representative" is a difficult task for a reviewer. With the current deluge of research and publications in the health field, few investigators have sufficient resources to conduct exhaustive reviews on common topics. Consequently it is important, at the very least, to attempt to define a universe of information sources on a topic, and then to establish meaningful priorities regarding that fraction of the universe to be screened within the available resources of a given review. This book provides a rather well defined "search denominator" and describes the limits of the search completed within the allocated budget. The basic reference file contained in the book was produced by a team effort that effectively used on-line bibliographic retrieval methods. All articles were screened, classified, and coded by two readers to ensure the relevance of the material included.

In regard to the second criterion (validity), it is even more difficult for reviewers to provide a data base that is sound scientifically. Adequate review of original research reports requires the combined expertise of scientists who keep up with the subject-matter literature and scientists who follow the quantitative and methodological literature. Unless supported by a grant or a contract of more than the usual size, a reviewer often assumes the task of literature screening and validation on his or her own, a difficult if not impossible task. The research file in this book was validated by two readers, with discrepancies of judgment being discussed, or referred to a third validator for mediation. Of 611 citations screened, 78 proved relevant and valid. Of the 78, 13 were of exceptional heuristic validity, and 12 (plus 2 from a separate search) had unusual quantitative validity. The reported results of those studies have immediate implications for improving the health care of stroke patients.

In relation to the third criterion (replicability), it is also difficult to provide sufficient documentation in a review to permit replication by other reviewers. Most reviewers infer from the absence of a review methods section that this criterion is not important. It is my personal opinion that methodological specificity is as important in reviews as it is in primary-data research such as controlled clinical trials. The results of reviews may be applied directly to patient care more often than results of isolated research studies. This book provides a level of detail regarding both its literature search and its literature validation methods that goes a long way toward meeting the replicability criterion--a quantum leap beyond the documentation provided by most traditional reviews.

Another important feature of this review is the coding system used to facilitate rapid location of relevant subject matter in terms of content and methods. For example, original research studies or evaluative reviews can be readily identified, and special codes differentiate reports of experimental and descriptive research designs. Similarly, the subject content of each referenced document can be identified in terms of special interest areas (e.g., gerontology, mental health, and physical disabilities), care setting (e.g., inpatient, outpatient, and home), services provided (e.g., medical, psychiatric, and occupational therapy), and patient characteristics (e.g., age and group relationships). Finally, codes detail research methods in terms of the investigator's source of data, patient functions evaluated, and treatment areas studied (e.g., cognitive, psychosocial, and preventive). This concept coding offers a practical means for the reader to combine concepts to specifically identify the type of content or information required. For example, if one needed original longitudinal research reports on rehabilitation of geriatric patients with stroke, the combination of P-2, S-19, -34, and -35, and M-3 would be searched to determine if such reports were included.

Admittedly this work has limitations. As the initial validated review in a series to be produced by the Efficacy Data Project, it has required considerable pioneering effort. The results represent a reasonable first product, and undoubtedly much has been learned to improve subsequent publications. What is most important, however, is the fact that AOTA made the policy decision to try to cope with what may be the key issue of the coming decade in the applied health sciences, namely, science information management. By establishing a base of valid information on topics of special relevance, particularly the impact of occupational therapy and related disciplines on improving health outcomes and cost savings, AOTA is making a substantial contribution to professional knowledge in general and patient care in particular.

John W. Williamson, MD
Associate Chief of Staff for Education,
  Veterans Administration Medical
  Center, Salt Lake City, Utah
Director of Health Services Research
  and Development Field Program,
  Veterans Administration Region 5

# ACKNOWLEDGMENTS

The Quality Assurance Division has relied on the talents of many staff, consultants, and volunteers to accomplish the tasks set before it in the stroke component of the Efficacy Data Project. On behalf of the American Occupational Therapy Association, I want to acknowledge and thank all of them.

The project consultant, John W. Williamson, brought to the effort his extensive skill as a theoretician, educator, and researcher devoted to improving the outcomes and the quality of health care. He also contributed his experience with a similar project on a far larger scale.

The actual substance of this book was the work of many people, as the Contents page attests. Susan M. Cotten conducted the pilot literature search to demonstrate the extent and the quality of the research available. Susan C. Merrill, who authored the qualitative synthesis, was the first project specialist. She ably and nearly singlehandedly ran the operation in its formative months. Her efforts were supported by Quality Assurance Division staff member Barbara E. Joe, who, along with coauthoring the Introduction, critiqued parts of the manuscript and assisted in other ways.

Susan Merrill was succeeded by Deborah Lieberman, who brought her fine coordinating skills and editing talents to the position of project specialist. Under her management the procedures for review were revised and expanded and the cohesiveness of the project maintained.

Kathy L. Kaplan assisted Deborah, and, having demonstrated her capabilities as an abstractor, followed Deborah as project specialist for the last few months of work on the stroke component. Deborah, Kathy, and two other able women, Mary C. Lawlor and Maureen Altobello, shared the abstracting responsibilities. The abstractors had the exacting task of editing or rewriting the abstracts originally published with the articles into summaries suitable for the Efficacy Data Project. Deborah and Kathy also had the difficult and demanding assignment of coding the abstracts.

Kenneth J. Ottenbacher made an especially valuable contribution in quantitatively synthesizing selected studies. The work of a careful, disciplined researcher is evident throughout his piece.

The twenty-four learned professionals whose names appear in the list following these acknowledgments reviewed articles for validity. The time they volunteered for this task was an important professional contribution. Two of them, Richard C. Cox and Wayne P. Pierson, were especially generous of their time, drawing on their broad experience in statistics and research design to review articles when previous reviewers disagreed.

The support of librarian Amy R. Bridgman was invaluable. She advised us on conducting the searches and tracked down many an elusive article.

On the administrative end of the Efficacy Data Project, Sue Ann Ketchum applied her organizational skills to the creation of a system for retrieving and fielding articles and for logging in the work of abstractors and reviewers. Jane E. King, Julie C. Anderson, and Catherine E. Skinner competently typed successive drafts of the manuscript.

Finally, in a highly professional manner, Margo Johnson brought all of the elements together into a unified whole, and Susan Hankoff gave the cover and the text the distinctive, appealing look they bear.

Patricia C. Ostrow, MA, OTR, FAOTA
Director, Quality Assurance Division,
American Occupational Therapy
Association

## EFFICACY DATA PROJECT
## REVIEW PANEL

Bette R. Bonder, PhD, OTR
Richard C. Cox, PhD
Charles Christiansen, EdD,
 OTR, FAOTA
Nancy B. Ellis, PhD, OTR,
 FAOTA
Grace E. Gilkeson, EdD,
 OTR, FAOTA
Lillian R. Greenstein, PhD,
 OTR, FAOTA
Ruth M. Griffin, PhD, OTR
Haru Hirama, EdD, OTR/L
Margot C. Howe, EdD, OTR,
 FAOTA
Jerry A. Johnson, EdD, OTR,
 FAOTA
Deborah Labovitz, PhD, OTR
Ruth Levine, EdD, OTR

Letitia P. Libman, PhD, OTR
Lela A. Llorens, PhD, OTR,
 FAOTA
William C. Mann, PhD, OTR
Marlys Mitchell, PhD, OTR,
 FAOTA
Laurence N. Peake, PhD, OTR,
 FAOTA
Wayne P. Pierson, PhD, OTR
Kathlyn L. Reed, PhD, OTR,
 FAOTA
Joan C. Rogers, PhD, OTR,
 FAOTA
Jacqueline M. Royce, PhD,
 OTR
Jane P. Rues, EdD, OTR
Kilulu Von Prince, EdD, OTR
Virginia White, EdD, OTR

# INTRODUCTION

*Patricia C. Ostrow, MA, OTR, FAOTA*
*Barbara E. Joe, MA*

The purpose of this resource book on the outcomes of stroke rehabilitation is to effect the orderly transmission of research findings into the practice of occupational therapy. This purpose is accomplished by presenting abstracts of research reports that were carefully screened for inclusion and by offering syntheses of selected studies that focus on the implications of the findings for occupational therapy.

The effort represented by this book is a circumscribed response to the overall need to establish a system for information management and dissemination in occupational therapy. The lack of such a system in most areas of health care creates an unnecessarily large gap between research and its practical application. A parallel need in chemistry and physics led the U.S. Congress to establish twenty-one data centers around the country to ensure access to relevant, valid, up-to-date information for practitioners of the physical sciences. Such a system is seen as an important precedent for consideration in the health care field (1).

The need for relevant and valid information and data in making health care decisions is great. Occupational therapy personnel, as well as all other health care practitioners, could improve their services if they had a greater awareness of research findings. Research information on the efficacy of occupational therapy is needed for many reasons. First, third-party payers frequently request data on treatment outcomes to justify the coverage of occupational therapy services. This is especially true in the current era of growing competition due to limited resources for health care. Second, therapists-in-training need research findings on outcomes to help them understand what the results of treatment may be. Third, data on the outcomes of treatment are the best source of information for establishing quality assurance standards to aid in the assessment of care. Finally, research on outcomes keeps occupational therapists abreast of new developments that may call for modifications in treatment procedures. Practice, representing the point at which clinician and patient/client come together, is the focus for all other concerns. If research is to have any meaningful impact, it must ultimately influence the course of patient/client care.

To have a practical effect on patient/client care, information on the efficacy of occupational therapy must be accessible, relevant, and valid. In terms of accessibility the sheer volume of health care literature is overwhelming to occupational therapy personnel seeking information on a particular subject. In 1985 there were approximately 8,500 U.S. health care journals and approximately

15,000 biomedical journals printed in English. Only 2,716 of these were listed in *Index Medicus* (based on reference no. 2, Table 2, p. 12, and information communicated by the National Library of Medicine, March 1985). Finding material pertinent to occupational therapy is even more difficult. Relatively few studies concentrate primarily on occupational therapy, and fewer still have *occupational therapy* in their title or as a key phrase.

As for relevance, studies, once found, are not necessarily applicable to practice. A physician-led evaluation of MEDLARS (Medical Literature Analysis and Retrieval System) for three well-known health conditions yielded 2,696 citations. Of a sample of 365 articles retrieved and analyzed, only 37 percent were in some way applicable to practice, and only 4 percent met criteria of information maturity for either quality assurance or clinical practice (1).

Finally, there is the problem of validity. The search for data relevant to occupational therapy treatment outcomes is further complicated because in many studies the conclusions are based on methodologically flawed, poorly reported research. The reliability and the validity of such studies must be seriously questioned. An early critical review of 295 research reports, including 149 analytic studies from ten leading medical journals, found that in "73% of the [analytic] reports read, conclusions were drawn when the justification for these conclusions was invalid" (3, p 148).

To meet the challenges of accessibility, relevance, and validity with specific regard to occupational therapy data, the American Occupational Therapy Association (AOTA) has developed the Efficacy Data Project. It is a continuing information management program pinpointing research that describes occupational-therapy-related treatment outcomes. Its goal is the orderly transmission of information about research relevant to the efficacy and the effectiveness of occupational therapy, making the information available for quality assurance studies, advocacy action, practice, and education. This book is on the project's first topic, stroke, chosen because it is the most frequent diagnosis encountered by practicing occupational therapy personnel (4).

A word about efficacy. It refers to "the extent to which a health care intervention can be shown to be beneficial under optimal conditions of care" (5, p 10). Sometimes efficacy as revealed in research is great, sometimes slight, sometimes nonexistent. Conceivably a health care intervention could be not only inefficacious but, in fact, harmful. Knowing the actual effects of care as revealed by research is important, whether they be good, bad, or indifferent. Occupational therapy personnel need to know what methods research has shown will not work, as well as what it has shown will work, in order to revise their services and sharpen their own observations. It is also important to understand the limits of research and to realize that an intervention may be less or more effective in a particular practice setting than it is under research conditions. However, research does show what can be achieved and thus provides a standard toward which to work.

# REVIEW METHOD
## SEARCHING THE LITERATURE

Stroke rehabilitation--defined as a comprehensive program to achieve improved health and welfare and the maximum physical, social, psychological, and vocational activity--is by its very nature pertinent to occupational therapy personnel. The emphasis of the literature search was stroke rehabilitation outcome studies or studies clarifying factors highly relevant to outcomes. Critical reviews of research, news articles, editorials, and correspondence on this subject were also included. All items had to have been published in or translated into the English language.

A variety of sources were used to identify possibilities. An initial search was made of Medline (a data base of journal citations on clinical medicine; part of MEDLARS), using the following descriptors: *stroke, cerebrovascular accident, hemiplegia, rehabilitation, splint,* and *activities of daily living,* along with *outcome assessment, clinical trials,* and *length of stay.* Other data bases such as CATLINE (Catalog on Line, covering books) and the *Cumulative Index to the American Journal of Occupational Therapy* were searched. A number of experts in the field of stroke rehabilitation, both physicians and therapists, were consulted. Prominent, recognized textbooks on stroke, some named in the reference lists of articles, some indexed in the card catalog of AOTA and the National Library of Medicine, were examined for citations. All major resources were tapped. The articles retrieved were subsequently examined for their own citations, creating a widening pyramid. Bibliographies and clearinghouses were investigated, such as the National Rehabilitation Information Center Bibliography and the National Health Standards and Quality Information Clearinghouse. A detailed description of the search is on file in the Quality Assurance Division.

In general, the search covered the period from 1976 through 1982, the latter being the year the Efficacy Data Project began. Some items are included even though they bear earlier dates.

Time and budget constraints also defined the parameters of the search, which was halted before all possible sources were exhausted. In June 1985, as this book was going into production, a search was conducted to identify relevant articles published since 1982. These are listed in the appendix.

## SCREENING THE LITERATURE FOR RELEVANCE AND VALIDITY

Following the search, the Quality Assurance Division staff screened all citations, abstracts, and documents for relevance to occupational therapy practice. To be considered relevant, an article had to be judged pertinent to the efficacy of occupational therapy in stroke treatment. Eighty-eight qualified.

These eighty-eight articles were sent to volunteer doctoral-level occupational therapists for review using a systematic screening protocol for scientific validity developed by the Quality Assurance Division in conjunction with John W. Williamson, MD, of Johns Hopkins University. The review criteria are available from the Quality Assurance Division. All articles were evaluated independently by two reviewers. In cases of disagreement about validity, or with studies involving complex statistical procedures, the articles were forwarded for final evaluation to Richard C. Cox, PhD, director of the Office for the Evaluation of Teaching, University of Pittsburgh, or to Wayne P. Pierson, PhD, OTR, chief of Research Consultation Services and deputy director of the Clinical Investigative Facility, USAF Medical Center, Lackland, Texas.

Ten articles were rejected in the screening because they did not meet the criteria for scientific adequacy. That left seventy-eight to be abstracted. Some articles reporting studies that may have had weak statistical results or flawed methodology have been included for their heuristic value. They were judged to present innovative concepts or developments that could have important implications for the field.

## SYNTHESIZING THE LITERATURE

To help the reader integrate the literature, both a qualitative synthesis and a quantitative synthesis were undertaken with selected studies. The methodology of each synthesis is described in its section.

# RESULTS

The studies selected for abstracting and synthesizing in this book do not, of course, give definitive detailed answers to occupational therapy personnel, dictating "Do this" and "Avoid that." Health care services can never be completely mechanical. Judgment and a wide range of variables, some of which cannot be controlled or quantified, will always influence the course of occupational therapy and health care treatment. However, the abstracts and the syntheses signal a direction and represent guides that recent literature offers. Examined as a whole, the abstracts point out the need for more research specifically directed toward the efficacy of occupational therapy in treating individuals with stroke. The syntheses distill some of the significant trends, questions, and conclusions from the literature. They lend credence to the value of stroke rehabilitation that includes occupational therapy, and they point out some of the variables that may be most relevant to successful outcomes.

## USING THIS BOOK

The text of this book is divided into three sections:

1. A collection of seventy-eight abstracts--abbreviated, accurate representations of the contents and the prominent features of the articles that were chosen for reporting. Selected comments of the reviewers have been included in paraphrased form. The abstracts are coded to guide the reader to those of particular interest. An explanation of the codes precedes the abstracts, as does a reference index listing all abstracts bearing the various codes.
2. A qualitative synthesis of thirteen articles selected as representative of key studies on the efficacy of occupational therapy practice with stroke patients.
3. A quantitative synthesis of fourteen articles selected using criteria related to the research design. Six articles covered in the two syntheses are the same. Two articles discussed in the quantitative synthesis were not in the original data base of eighty-eight and hence are not among those abstracted.

Occupational therapy personnel and others who want to know quickly the main conclusions of the book should read the qualitative synthesis and the abstract of the quantitative synthesis. Clinicians looking for many good ideas are advised to scan the abstracts. Ideas specific to a topic can be located by using the reference index. Scholars will find the quantitative synthesis particularly informative.

All readers may be interested in several Efficacy Data Briefs that are companions to this book. Prepared by the Quality Assurance Division, the briefs offer more extensive summaries of selected studies and fuller discussions of their significance. They

5

address the perspectives of administrators, legislators, and physicians, as well as occupational therapy personnel. The articles covered in data briefs are designated by notes following the abstracts.

## REFERENCES

1. Williamson JW: Information management in quality assurance. *Nurs Research* 29(2):78-82, 1980
2. *Coping with the Biomedical Literature Explosion: A Qualitative Approach.* New York: The Rockefeller Foundation, December 1978
3. Schor S, Karten I: Statistical evaluation of medical journal manuscripts. *JAMA* 195:145-150, 1966
4. *Member Data Surveys.* Rockville, MD: American Occupational Therapy Association, July 1982
5. Williamson JW: *Improving Medical Practice and Health Care.* Cambridge, MA: Ballinger, 1977

# GUIDES AND ABSTRACTS

*Deborah Lieberman, MA, OTR/L*
*Mary C. Lawlor, EdM, OTR*
*Maureen Altobello, BA*
*Kathy L. Kaplan, MS, OTR*

This section contains seventy-eight abstracts of articles related to the outcomes of stroke rehabilitation. Each abstract is coded to help readers rapidly and accurately identify the abstracts pertinent to their area of interest. The abstracts are preceded by a reference index, which lists under each code the numbers of all of the abstracts bearing that code. Using the reference index, readers may--

1. Review all of the abstracts listed under one code--for example, everything under S-21, indicating that occupational therapy services were provided.
2. Select several codes describing the information that they seek, and review all of the abstracts under each of those codes--for example, all of the abstracts under M-7 and M-13, evaluation and treatment related to skills and performance in activities of daily living.
3. Cross-index among several codes and review only the abstracts that appear under all of the codes--for example, abstracts under P-2, original research; S-1, physical disabilities; S-12, long-term care in a rehabilitation center; and S-34 and S-35, adults sixty-one to seventy-six and adults seventy-seven or more years old.

# EXPLANATION OF THE CODE

Articles have been coded by the following headings and subheadings:

P = Purpose--the author's reason for writing the document

T = Type--the major form the document takes

S = Subject--five subcategories that describe aspects of the study's subject matter:
- Special interest area--the major area of occupational therapy clinical practice
- Care setting--the location/type of the facility or the setting in which care was provided
- Services provided--the professions of the practitioners who administered treatment
- Patient/client characteristics--the age of the study population
- Sample or universe--the number of subjects involved in the study

M = Method--four subcategories that describe how the study was conducted, the areas studied relevant to occupational therapy, and the type of intervention used in the study
- Sources of data--where and how the information for the study was obtained
- Treatment areas--occupational therapy service categories adapted from AOTA's *Occupational Therapy Product Output Reporting System and Uniform Terminology for Reporting Occupational Therapy Services*
- Evaluation areas--categories similar to those under Treatment Areas
- Miscellaneous--additional items of interest related to the focus or the aim of the article.

Table 1 breaks this information down into specific descriptors and their corresponding codes.

Table 1
Headings, Descriptors, and Codes

| Purpose | Code |
|---|---|
| (Information Categories) | |
| State-of-the-science consensus: comprehensive, consensual analysis by expert panel--commission report, white paper, consensus statement, conference report | P-1 |
| Original research: a primary investigation or a reanalysis of data | P-2 |
| Evaluation review: objective judgmental analysis, critique, presentation of both sides of an issue | P-3 |
| Educational review: objective nonjudgmental review, test, exposition | P-4 |
| Opinion statement: subjective judgmental analysis, editorial, letter, essay, commentary | P-5 |
| Information resource: data table, manual, guidelines, proceedings, minutes | P-6 |
| News: brief factual report, objective commentary on recent events | P-7 |

Type

| | Code |
|---|---|
| Unpublished report | T-1 |
| Research | |
| Descriptive: a report of a situation, a phenomenon, people; a case study; a survey | T-2 |
| Experimental: a report of a cause-effect relationship between variables, truly experimental,quasi-experimental, or preexperimental; factoral designs | T-3 |
| Ex post facto: a description of differences between two nonrandomly selected groups, after the fact | T-4 |
| Correlational: a report of the degree of relationship among two or more variables | T-5 |
| Analytic or comparative: an analysis of a particular situation, a comparison of two or more study situations | T-6 |
| Report of a model, a method, a pilot study, a program | T-7 |
| Conference seminar or symposium proceedings | T-8 |
| Editorial, philosophical statement | T-9 |
| Manual, booklet, organization report | T-10 |
| Review, history | T-11 |
| Bibliography | T-12 |
| Annotated bibliography | T-13 |

Subject

| | |
|---|---|
| **Special interest area** | |
| Physical disabilities | S-1 |
| Gerontology | S-2 |
| Mental health | S-3 |
| Sensory integration | S-4 |
| Developmental disabilities | S-5 |
| **Care setting** | |
| Inpatient, general | S-6 |
| Inpatient, acute care | S-7 |
| Inpatient, university medical center | S-8 |
| Inpatient, state facility | S-9 |
| Home care | S-10 |
| Long-term care, inpatient | S-11 |
| Long-term care, rehabilitation center | S-12 |
| Long-term care, nursing home | S-13 |
| Long-term care, skilled nursing facility | S-14 |
| Outpatient, community based | S-15 |
| Outpatient, hospital based | S-16 |
| **Services provided** | |
| Medical | S-17 |
| Psychiatry/psychology | S-18 |
| Rehabilitation | S-19 |
| Vocational rehabilitation | S-20 |
| Occupational therapy | S-21 |
| Physical therapy | S-22 |
| Social work | S-23 |
| Speech therapy | S-24 |
| Recreational therapy | S-25 |
| Expressive arts (art, dance, music) | S-26 |
| Activity therapy | S-27 |
| **Patient/client characteristics** | |
| Infant--0-23 months old | S-28 |
| Child--2-12 years old | S-29 |
| Adolescent--13-17 years old | S-30 |
| Adult below 30 years old | S-31 |
| Adult 30-45 years old | S-32 |
| Adult 46-60 years old | S-33 |
| Adult 61-76 years old | S-34 |
| Adult 77 or more years old | S-35 |
| **Sample or universe** | |
| Individual in a role within a group | S-36 |
| Pair of interrelated group members (dyad) | S-37 |
| Primary group (20 or less) | S-38 |
| Secondary group (21 or more) | S-39 |
| Tertiary group (crowd, public, etc.--100) | S-40 |
| State, nation, society | S-41 |

## Method

Sources of data
    Primary data on patients/clients (direct observation,      M-1
        questionnaire, interview, test, rating scale,
        inventory)
    Secondary data on patients/clients (medical record,      M-2
        therapist's chart)
    Longitudinal or follow-up study      M-3
    Estimated data      M-4
    Published paper or abstract      M-5
    No specific information source      M-6
Evaluation areas
    Independent living/daily living skill and      M-7
        performance
    Sensorimotor skill and performance      M-8
    Cognitive skill and performance      M-9
    Psychosocial skill and performance      M-10
    Therapeutic adaptation      M-11
    Specialized      M-12
Treatment areas
    Independent living/daily living skill:  physical,      M-13
        psychological/emotional, work, play/leisure
    Sensorimotor component      M-14
    Cognitive component      M-15
    Psychosocial component      M-16
    Therapeutic adaptation      M-17
    Prevention      M-18
Miscellaneous
    Cost      M-19
    Administration      M-20
    Quality assurance      M-21

# REFERENCE INDEX

S-9--Care Setting: Inpatient,
State Facility
72

S-10--Care Setting: Home
Care
11, 33, 37, 63, 65, 76

S-11--Care Setting: Long-
Term Care, Inpatient
16, 30, 31, 41, 42, 55

S-12--Care Setting: Long-
Term Care, Rehabilitation
Center
1, 2, 3, 8, 9, 15, 17, 19, 20,
21, 22, 23, 24, 25, 27, 32,
36, 40, 43, 44, 45, 46, 47,
48, 50, 51, 52, 57, 59, 61,
67, 68, 74, 75

S-14--Care Setting: Long-
Term Care, Skilled Nursing
Facility
35

S-15--Care Setting:
Outpatient, Community Based
6, 7, 18, 61

S-16--Care Setting:
Outpatient, Hospital Based
20, 34, 38, 62, 63, 77

S-18--Services Provided:
Psychiatry/Psychology
9, 45

S-19--Services Provided:
Rehabilitation
1, 2, 3, 4, 5, 6, 10, 11, 13,
15, 17, 19, 20, 21, 22, 23,
24, 25, 26, 27, 28, 30, 31,
32, 33, 35, 36, 39, 41, 42,
43, 46, 47, 48, 49, 50, 51,

52, 54, 56, 57, 59, 62, 65,
67, 68, 69, 70, 73, 76

S-20--Services Provided:
Vocational Rehabilitation
75

S-21--Services Provided:
Occupational Therapy
8, 12, 29, 34, 37, 55, 60, 61,
63, 64, 66, 71, 74

S-22--Services Provided:
Physical Therapy
11, 12, 14, 16, 29, 38, 40,
58, 63, 64, 77

S-24--Services Provided:
Speech Therapy
29, 63

S-33--Patient/Client
Characteristics: Adult 46-60
Years Old
1, 2, 4, 6, 7, 8, 15, 40, 43,
47, 67, 68, 75, 76, 77

S-34--Patient/Client
Characteristics: Adult 61-76
Years Old
2, 3, 5, 7, 9, 10, 11, 16, 17,
18, 21, 22, 23, 24, 25, 26,
27, 28, 29, 30, 31, 32, 33,
34, 35, 37, 38, 41, 42, 44,
45, 46, 48, 50, 51, 52, 54,
56, 57, 61, 62, 63, 64, 65,
70, 71, 72, 73, 74, 76

S-36--Sample or Universe:
Individual in a Role Within a
Group
35, 37, 38, 43

S-38--Sample or Universe:
Primary Group (20 or Less)
12, 39, 66, 71

S-39--Sample or Universe:
Secondary Group (21 or
More)
1, 6, 7, 11, 16, 18, 26, 32,
34, 40, 42, 44, 45, 55, 56,
59, 67, 68, 75, 76, 77

S-40--Sample or Universe:
Tertiary Group (Crowd,
Public, etc.--100)
2, 3, 4, 5, 8, 9, 10, 15, 17,
21, 22, 23, 24, 25, 27, 28,
29, 30, 31, 33, 36, 41, 46,
47, 48, 49, 50, 51, 52, 54,
61, 62, 63, 64, 65, 70, 72,
73, 74

S-41--Sample or Universe:
State, Nation, Society
19, 57

M-1--Sources of Data:
Primary Data on
Patients/Clients
1, 2, 3, 4, 6, 7, 8, 9, 10, 12,
16, 17, 18, 21, 23, 25, 26,
27, 29, 30, 31, 32, 33, 34,
37, 38, 39, 40, 41, 42, 43,
44, 45, 46, 47, 48, 50, 53,
54, 55, 56, 57, 59, 61, 63,
65, 66, 67, 68, 69, 71, 73,
74, 76, 77

M-2--Sources of Data:
Secondary Data on
Patients/Clients
2, 11, 24, 36, 49, 52, 64, 70,
72, 75

M-3--Sources of Data:
Longitudinal or Follow-up
Study
15, 28, 46, 51

M-5--Sources of Data:
Published Paper or Abstract
14, 19, 20, 35, 58, 69, 78

M-6--Sources of Data: No
Specific Information Source
13, 60

M-7--Evaluation Areas:
Independent Living/Daily
Living Skill and Performance
1, 2, 3, 4, 6, 7, 8, 9, 10, 11,
15, 16, 17, 18, 20, 21, 23,
24, 25, 26, 27, 28, 29, 30,
31, 32, 33, 35, 36, 37, 40,
41, 42, 43, 44, 45, 46, 47,
48, 49, 50, 51, 52, 53, 54,
56, 57, 59, 61, 62, 63, 64,
65, 67, 68, 69, 70, 72, 73,
74, 75, 76, 77

M-8--Evaluation Areas:
Sensorimotor Skill and
Performance
2, 5, 6, 8, 10, 12, 14, 15, 16,
17, 18, 21, 23, 24, 25, 26,
30, 32, 33, 34, 35, 37, 38,
39, 40, 41, 42, 44, 45, 47,
48, 49, 50, 51, 53, 57, 59,
61, 62, 63, 64, 67, 68, 69,
70, 71, 72, 73, 74, 75, 77,
78

M-9--Evaluation Areas:
Cognitive Skill and
Performance
9, 15, 17, 18, 23, 25, 26, 27,
32, 33, 42, 44, 45, 48, 59,
62, 64, 69, 75

M-10--Evaluation Areas:
Psychosocial Skill and
Performance
4, 6, 7, 15, 17, 18, 28, 31,
32, 33, 38, 43, 46, 48, 49,
51, 54, 69, 76

M-11--Evaluation Areas:
Therapeutic Adaptation
6, 12, 39, 51, 55, 58, 65, 66,
70

M-13--Treatment Areas:
Independent Living/Daily
Living Skill: Physical,
Psychological/Emotional,
Work, Play/Leisure
1, 5, 8, 10, 13, 16, 17, 20,
21, 22, 29, 30, 31, 35, 40,
41, 42, 43, 49, 50, 52, 53,
54, 57, 63, 64, 65, 68, 76

M-14--Treatment Areas:
Sensorimotor Component
5, 8, 10, 12, 13, 14, 16, 21,
22, 29, 34, 35, 38, 40, 42,
43, 49, 50, 53, 57, 60, 63,
64, 67, 68, 71, 72, 77, 78

M-16--Treatment Areas:
Psychosocial Component
13, 22, 31, 41, 43

M-17--Treatment Areas:
Therapeutic Adaptation
5, 12, 29, 30, 35, 37, 39, 58,
65, 66

M-18--Treatment Areas:
Prevention
65

M-19--Miscellaneous: Cost
3, 11,19, 20, 21, 25, 36, 47

M-20--Miscellaneous:
Administration
11, 36

M-21--Quality Assurance
3, 4

15

# BIBLIOGRAPHY OF ABSTRACTED ARTICLES

1. Andersen AL, Hanvik LJ, Brown JR: A statistical analysis of rehabilitation in hemiplegia. *Geriatrics* 5:214-218, 1950
2. Anderson E, Anderson TP, Kottke FJ: Stroke rehabilitation: Maintenance of achieved gains. *Arch Phys Med Rehab* 58:345-352, 1977
3. Anderson TP, Baldridge M, Ettinger MG: Quality of care for completed stroke without rehabilitation: Evaluation by assessing patient outcomes. *Arch Phys Med Rehab* 60:103-107, 1979
4. Anderson TP, McClure WJ, Athelstan G, Anderson E, Crewe N, Arndts L, Ferguson MB, Baldridge M, Gullickson G, Kottke FJ: Stroke rehabilitation: Evaluation of its quality by assessing patient outcomes. *Arch Phys Med Rehab* 59:170-175, 1978
5. Andrews K, Brocklehurst JC, Richards B, Laycock PJ: The rate of recovery from stroke--and its measurement. *Int Rehab Med* 3:155-161, 1981
6. Belcher SA, Clowers MR, Cabanayan AC: Independent living rehabilitation needs of postdischarge stroke persons: A pilot study. *Arch Phys Med Rehab* 59:404-409, 1978
7. Belcher SA, Clowers MR, Cabanayan AC, Fordyce WE: Activity patterns of married and single individuals after stroke. *Arch Phys Med Rehab* 63:308-312, 1982
8. Bell E, Jurek K, Wilson T: Hand skill measurement: A gauge for treatment. *Am J Occup Ther* 30:80-86, 1976
9. Bourestom NC, Howard MT: Behavioral correlates of recovery of self-care in hemiplegic patients. *Arch Phys Med Rehab* 49:449-454, 1968
10. Brocklehurst JC, Andrews K, Richards B, Laycock PJ: How much physical therapy for patients with stroke? *Br Med J* 279:1307-1310, 1978
11. Bryant NH, Candland L, Loewenstein R: Comparison of care and cost outcomes for stroke patients with and without home care. *Stroke* 5:54-59, 1974
12. Charait SE: A comparison of volar and dorsal splinting of the hemiplegic hand. *Am J Occup Ther* 22:319-321, 1968
13. Chaudhuri G: Rehabilitation of the stroke patient. *Geriatrics* 35:45-46, 49-50, 54; 1980
14. Chin PL: Physical techniques in stroke rehabilitation. *J Royal College of Physicians of London* 16:165-169, 1982
15. Coughlan AK, Humphrey M: Presenile stroke: Long-term

outcome for patients and their families. *Rheumatology and Rehab* 21:115-122, 1982

16. Denes G, Semenza C, Stoppa E, Lis A: Unilateral spatial neglect and recovery from hemiplegia: A follow-up study. *Brain* 105:543-552, 1982

17. Diller L, Buxbaum J, Chiotelis S: Relearning motor skills in hemiplegia: Error analysis. *Genet Psychol Monographs* 85:249-286, 1972

18. Feibel JH, Springer CJ: Depression and failure to resume social activities after stroke. *Arch Phys Med Rehab* 63:276-278, 1982

19. Feigenson JS: Stroke rehabilitation: Effectiveness, benefits, and cost. Some practical considerations (editorial). *Stroke* 10:1-4, 1979

20. Feigenson JS: Stroke rehabilitation: Outcome studies and guidelines for alternative levels of care. *Stroke* 12:372-375, 1981

21. Feigenson JS, Gitlow HS, Greenberg SD: The disability oriented rehabilitation unit--A major factor influencing stroke outcome. *Stroke* 10:5-8, 1979

22. Feigenson JS, McCarthy ML: Stroke rehabilitation, part 2: Guidelines for establishing a stroke rehabilitation unit. *NY State J Med*, Aug 1977, pp 1430-1434

23. Feigenson JS, McCarthy ML, Greenberg SD, Feigenson WD: Factors influencing outcome and length of stay in a stroke rehabilitation unit, part 2: Comparison of 318 screened and 248 unscreened patients. *Stroke* 8:657-662, 1977

24. Feigenson JS, McCarthy ML, Meese PD, Feigenson WD, Greenberg SD, Rubin E, McDowell FH: Stroke rehabilitation, part 1: Factors predicting outcome and length of stay--an overview. *NY State J Med*, Aug 1977, pp 1426-1430

25. Feigenson JS, McDowell FH, Meese P, McCarthy ML, Greenberg SD: Factors influencing outcome and length of stay in a stroke rehabilitation unit, part 1: Analysis of 248 unscreened patients--medical and functional prognostic indicators. *Stroke* 8:651-656, 1977

26. Feldman DJ, Lee PR, Unterecker J, Lloyd K, Rusk HA, Toole A: A comparison of functionally oriented medical care and formal rehabilitation in the management of patients with hemiplegia due to cerebrovascular disease. *J Chron Dis* 15:297-310, 1962

27. Forer SK, Miller LS: Rehabilitation outcome: Comparative analysis of different patient types. *Arch Phys Med Rehab* 61:359-365, 1980

28. Garraway WM, Akhtar AJ, Hockey L, Prescott RJ:

Management of acute stroke in the elderly: Follow-up of a controlled trial. *Br Med J* 281:827-829, 1980

29. Garraway WM, Akhtar AJ, Prescott RJ, Hockey L: Management of acute stroke in the elderly: Preliminary results of a controlled trial. *Br Med J* 280:1040-1043, 1980

30. Garraway WM, Akhtar AJ, Smith DL, Smith ME: The triage of stroke rehabilitation. *J Epidemiology and Community Health* 35:39-44, 1981

31. Garraway WM, Walton MS, Akhtar AJ, Prescott RJ: The use of health and social services in the management of stroke in the community: Results from a controlled trial. *Age and Ageing* 10:95-104, 1981

32. Gordon EE, Kohn KH: Evaluation of rehabilitation methods in the hemiplegic patient. *J Chron Dis* 19:3-16, 1966

33. Granger CV, Sherwood CC, Greer DS: Functional status measures in a comprehensive stroke care program. *Arch Phys Med Rehab* 58:555-561, 1977

34. Greenberg S, Fowler RS Jr: Kinesthetic biofeedback: A treatment modality for elbow range of motion in hemiplegia. *Am J Occup Ther* 34:738-743, 1980

35. Gresham GE: Rehabilitation of the geriatric patient: Stroke rehabilitation, the rehabilitation team, and the usefulness of functional assessment. *Primary Care* 9:239-247, 1982

36. Harasymiw SJ, Albrecht GL: Admission and discharge indicators as aids in optimizing comprehensive rehabilitation services. *Scand J Rehab Med* 11:123-128, 1979

37. Harrison H: The role of the pressure splint in sensory stimulation of the hemiplegic upper extremity. *North Carolina Occupational Therapy Association Selected Papers,* Oct 1982, pp 8-14

38. Honer J, Mohr T, Roth R: Electromyographic biofeedback to dissociate an upper extremity synergy pattern: A case report. *Phys Ther* 62:299-303, 1982

39. Hurd MM, Farrell KH, Waylonis GW: Shoulder sling for hemiplegia: Friend or foe? *Arch Phys Med Rehab* 55:519-522, 1974

40. Inaba M, Edberg E, Montgomery J, Gillis MK: Effectiveness of functional training, active exercise, and resistive exercise for patients with hemiplegia. *Phys Ther* 53:28-35, 1973

41. Isaacs B: Five years' experience of a stroke unit. *Health Bull* 35:94-98, 1979

42. Isaacs B, Marks R: Determinants of outcome of stroke rehabilitation. *Age and Ageing* 2:139-149, 1973

43. Jain S: Operant conditioning for management of a

noncompliant rehabilitation case after stroke. *Arch Phys Med Rehab* 63:374-376, 1982

44. Kaplan J, Hier DB: Visuospatial deficits after right hemisphere stroke. *Am J Occup Ther* 36:314-321, 1982

45. Kinsella G, Ford B: Acute recovery patterns in stroke patients: Neuropsychological factors. *Med J Australia* 2:663-666, 1980

46. Labi MLC, Phillips TF, Gresham GE: Psychosocial disability in physically restored long-term stroke survivors. *Arch Phys Med Rehab* 61:561-565, 1980

47. Lehmann JF, DeLateur BJ, Fowler RS Jr, Warren CG, Arnhold R, Schertzer G, Hurka R, Whitmore JJ, Masock AJ, Chambers KH: Stroke: Does rehabilitation affect outcome? *Arch Phys Med Rehab* 56:375-382, 1975

48. Lehmann JF, DeLateur BJ, Fowler RS Jr, Warren CG, Arnhold R, Schertzer G, Hurka R, Whitmore JJ, Masock AJ, Chambers KH: Stroke rehabilitation: Outcome and prediction. *Arch Phys Med Rehab* 56:383-389, 1975

49. McCann BC, Culbertson RA: Comparison of two systems for stroke rehabilitation in a general hospital. *J Am Geriatrics Soc* 24:211-216, 1976

50. McClatchie G: Survey of the rehabilitation outcome of strokes. *Med J Australia* 1:649-651, 1980

51. Moskowitz E, Lightbody FEH, Freitag NS: Long-term follow-up of the poststroke patient. *Arch Phys Med Rehab* 53:167-172, 1972

52. Mossman PL, Kerr M, Stever R: Hospital utilization in the rehabilitation of completed stroke. *Minnesota Med,* Jul 1977, pp 498-502

53. Muller EA: Influence of training and of inactivity on muscle strength. *Arch Phys Med Rehab* 51:449-462, 1970

54. Murray SK, Garraway WM, Akhtar AJ, Prescott RJ: Communication between home and hospital in the management of acute stroke in the elderly: Results from a controlled trial. *Health Bull* 40:214-219, 1982

55. Neuhaus BE, Ascher ER, Coullon BA, Donohue MV, Einbond A, Glover JM, Goldberg SR, Takai VL: A survey of rationales for and against hand splinting in hemiplegia. *Am J Occup Ther* 35:83-90, 1981

56. Pendarvis JF, Grinnell RM Jr: The use of a rehabilitation team for stroke patients. *Social Work in Health Care* 6:77-85, 1980

57. Redford JB, Harris JD: Rehabilitation of the elderly stroke patient. *Amer Family Physician* 22:153-160, 1980

58. Robins V, Braun RM, Voss DE: Should patients with hemiplegia wear a sling? *Phys Ther* 49:1029-1030, 1969

59. Rosenthal AM, Pearson L, Medenica B, Manaster A, Smith CS: Correlation of perceptual factors with rehabilitation of hemiplegic patients. *Arch Phys Med Rehab* 46:461-466, 1965

60. Shah S: Occupational therapy for motor re-education of hemiplegics. In *Proceedings of the 2nd International Congress on Muscle Diseases,* BA Kakulas, Editor. Amsterdam, The Netherlands: Excerpta Medica, 1971, part 2, pp 682-685

61. Shah SK, Corones J: Volition following hemiplegia. *Arch Phys Med Rehab* 61:523-528, 1980

62. Sheikh K, Meade TW, Brennan PJ, Goldenberg E, Smith DS: Intensive rehabilitation after stroke: Service implications. *Community Med* 3:210-216, 1981

63. Smith DS, Goldenberg E, Ashburn A, Kinsella G, Sheikh K, Brennan PJ, Meade TW, Zutshi DW, Perry JD, Reeback JS: Remedial therapy after stroke: A randomized controlled trial. *Br Med J* 282:517-520, 1981

64. Smith ME, Garraway WM, Smith DL, Akhtar AJ: Therapy impact on functional outcome in a controlled trial of stroke rehabilitation. *Arch Phys Med Rehab* 63:21-24, 1982

65. Smith ME, Walton MS, Garraway WM: The use of aids and adaptations in a study of stroke rehabilitation. *Health Bull* 39:98-106, 1981

66. Snook JH: Spasticity reduction splint. *Am J Occup Ther* 33:648-651, 1979

67. Stern PH, McDowell F, Miller JM, Robinson M: Effects of facilitation exercise techniques in stroke rehabilitation. *Arch Phys Med Rehab* 51:526-531, 1970

68. Stern PH, McDowell F, Miller JM, Robinson M: Factors influencing stroke rehabilitation. *Stroke* 2:213-218, 1971

69. Stonnington HH: Rehabilitation in cerebrovascular diseases. *Primary Care* 7:87-106, 1980

70. Tan ES, Don RG: Rehabilitation of cerebrovascular disease with neurological deficits--results of 500 cases treated between 1973 & 1978. *Singapore Med J* 22:210-213, 1981

71. Trombly CA: Effects of selected activities on finger extension of adult hemiplegic patients. *Am J Occup Ther* 18:233-239, 1964

72. Truscott BL, Kretschmann CM, Toole JF, Pajak TF: Early rehabilitative care in community hospitals: Effect on quality of survivorship following a stroke. *Stroke* 5:623-629, 1974

73. Wade DT, Skilbeck CE, Hewer RL: Predicting Barthel ADL score at 6 months after an acute stroke. *Arch Phys Med Rehab* 64:24-27, 1983

74. Warren M: Relationship of constructional apraxia and body scheme disorders to dressing performance in adult CVA. *Am J Occup Ther* 35:431-437, 1981
75. Weisbroth S, Esibill N, Zuger RR: Factors in the vocational success of hemiplegic patients. *Arch Phys Med Rehab* 52:441-446, 486; 1971
76. Wolcott LE, Wheeler PC, Ballard P, Crumb CK, Miles G, Mueller A: Home-care vs. institutional rehabilitation of stroke: A comparative study. *Missouri Med* 63:722-724, 1966
77. Wolf SL, Baker MP, Kelly JL: EMG biofeedback in stroke: A 1-year follow-up on the effect of patient characteristics. *Arch Phys Med Rehab* 61:351-355, 1980
78. Yu J: Functional recovery with and without training following brain damage in experimental animals: A review. *Arch Phys Med Rehab* 57:38-41, 1976

# ABSTRACTS

**1**  Andersen AL, Hanvik LJ, Brown JR

CODES:
P-2; T-6; S-1,
12, 19, 33,
39; M-1, 7, 13

## A STATISTICAL ANALYSIS OF REHABILITATION IN HEMIPLEGIA

*Geriatrics* 5:214-218, 1950

Data on eighty-two stroke patients treated by the Rehabilitation Service of the Minneapolis Veterans Administration Hospital in 1949 were analyzed to assess the effectiveness of the rehabilitation therapy program. Patients were grouped by age, over or under fifty-five years; by the interval between onset and treatment, over or under three months; and by the site of their disability, left or right hemiplegia. The treatment program was designed for each patient in accordance with the results of a complete evaluation, including medical, neurological, and psychological examinations and a social and vocational evaluation. A physician supervised the treatment. The etiology of the hemiplegia and the complicating conditions existing among the patients studied are described. Statistics and the scoring variables used in evaluating the progress of patients' rehabilitation are also included.

In general, the results indicated that greater efficiency in retraining was achieved when a patient was placed on a rehabilitation program as soon as possible after a disability was incurred. Also, younger patients had a better prognosis, apparently due to a greater incentive to achieve. Morale was a major factor in determining the length of rehabilitation and the ultimate degree of success. Patients with right hemiplegia had lower ambulation improvement scores and varied more in the length of time they spent on the rehabilitation service.

> ***Reviewers' Comments:*** The adequacy of the documentation and the supportability of the validity components are debatable. The study does offer some interesting ideas about the differences between
> (continued on next page)

younger and older patients, but the data seem too questionable to allow definitive conclusions. The article may have more relevance to program planning for comprehensive rehabilitation than to program planning for occupational therapy.

**2** Anderson E, Anderson TP, Kottke FJ

CODES:
P-2; T-4; S-1,
12, 19, 33, 34,
40; M-1, 2, 7, 8

# STROKE REHABILITATION: MAINTENANCE OF ACHIEVED GAINS

*Archives of Physical Medicine and Rehabilitation* 58:345-352, 1977

A retrospective study of patients who participated in a complete rehabilitation program between 1960 and 1970 was conducted. Of the 250 patients who were identified, 107 were living at the time of the study and could be located. Of these, 79 were available for home interview and chosen for the study population. Information on 109 deceased patients was used for portions of the analysis, yielding a total of 188 subjects (53 percent males and 47 percent females). The deceased group had a mean age at the onset of stroke of sixty-one years and a mean age at the time of death of sixty-six years. The surviving patients who were interviewed had a mean age of sixty years and a mean age at the onset of stroke of fifty years. Age differences between the two groups were not considered to be significant. The five measures of rehabilitative activity studied were self-care, mobility, amount of time spent at a major daily activity, vocational status, and overall rehabilitative status.

The independent variables that correlated positively with these rehabilitative functions were living at home rather than in a nursing home and having an accepting attitude about present status. The gains made during rehabilitation after stroke were maintained or improved by the majority of patients when assessed two to twelve years later. The gains were maintained throughout the long survival time, averaging seven to eight years. Additional loss, when it did occur, was usually secondary to a superimposed health problem.

> ***Reviewers' Comments:*** The article raises the issue of the importance of the patient's attitude and the family's inclusion in the rehabilitation program. Occupational therapy can assist, particularly in the training of family members.

**3** Anderson TP, Baldridge M, Ettinger MG

CODES:
P-2; T-4; S-1, 7,
21; M-1, 12, 19,
34, 40

# QUALITY OF CARE FOR COMPLETED STROKE WITHOUT REHABILITATION: EVALUATION BY ASSESSING PATIENT OUTCOMES

*Archives of Physical Medicine and Rehabilitation* 60:103-107, 1979

Further research was initiated as the result of a follow-up study of 119 patients with completed stroke who participated in a rehabilitation program at the University of Minnesota Hospitals. In the earlier study (see abstract no. 4) the Health Accounting method of quality assurance was used to measure and assess the health status of the patients. They were found to have achieved a health status better than originally anticipated by the study team. That finding raised questions about the outcomes for stroke patients who had not had rehabilitation.

In the present study a retrospective analysis of patient records at the Hennepin County Medical Center provided a second sample of 84 patients who had received little or no rehabilitation therapy following stroke. The untreated group was not matched with the group given rehabilitation, but its members were generally less severely involved, although older on the average. The goals of the study were to compare the outcomes of the two groups of stroke patients, only one of which had participated in a rehabilitation program; to test the method of Health Accounting in two situations for the same health problem; and to contribute to data on long-range outcomes and the quality of care provided to stroke patients. Outcomes were measured by telephone interview using a modified Functional Limitation Scale to record data. (Descriptions of the scale are included in the article.) The results were then compared with the previous study group of 119 patients. Of the original 84 untreated patients, 39 (42 percent) had died, which was slightly higher than had been estimated. Within this group 47 percent were capable of self-care, 56 percent lived at home, and 44 percent were institutionalized--all outcomes within established quality assurance limits. Although the rehabilitation patients had a 60-percent survival rate, only 2 percent better than the untreated group, 82 percent of the survivors were living independently, and 69 percent were independent in self-care. Only 18 percent were institutionalized.

Factors identified as contributing to the stroke patient's quality of life that can be enhanced by rehabilitation were independence in self-care; living at home or outside an institution; and involvement in employment, homemaking, or some type of daily activity. Although the modified scale used was not sensitive enough to measure these factors fully, it did reflect quality-of-life differences in general between stroke patients who experienced rehabilitation and those who did not.

The authors conclude that rehabilitation did not significantly lengthen the duration of survival from onset to interview or death, but it did positively affect the quality of life during survival. These results are too often discounted in measuring the costs of rehabilitation and its significance.

*Reviewers' Comments:* The adequacy of the validity components is at issue. There is strong evidence that the study groups were not homogeneous in age and socioeconomic status, and that prevents generalization of the conclusions. Also, some of the comparisons made between the groups are weak; thus, the study's internal validity is threatened. However, the study does provide supporting evidence for the role of

(continued on next page)

> rehabilitation in the quality of life following stroke and for a life span for stroke survivors sufficient to warrant rehabilitation intervention including occupational therapy.

**4** Anderson TP, McClure WJ, Athelstan G,
Anderson E, Crewe N, Arndts L,
Ferguson MB, Baldridge M, Gullickson G,
Kottke FJ

CODES:
P-2; T-7; S-1, 8,
19, 33, 40; M-1,
7, 10, 21

## STROKE REHABILITATION: EVALUATION OF ITS QUALITY BY ASSESSING PATIENT OUTCOMES

*Archives of Physical Medicine and Rehabilitation* 59:170-175, 1978

A systematic method for assessing the quality of rehabilitation for completed stroke using small-group estimation techniques (a modified version of an outcome-oriented quality assurance system) was evaluated. Estimates of outcomes developed by an interdisciplinary study team were compared with actual outcomes obtained from data in patient records and follow-up interviews. On the basis of their medical records 119 younger stroke patients met the criteria for inclusion in the study. They were aged twenty-one to sixty years at admission, between April 1, 1960, and December 31, 1972; were diagnosed as hemiplegic, hemiparetic, and/or aphasic; and received at least three weeks of inpatient care. Of the 73 living patients, 67 agreed to follow-up interviews. Data from these 67 patients formed the basis for study conclusions. Williamson's Functional Limitation Scale and items selected to measure changes in life-style, degree of dependence, and living costs provided the data used to grade patients. Patient status was scored at discharge, during the interval between discharge and follow-up, and at follow-up.

Outcomes were better than estimated: Standards had indicated that 29 percent of the patients should be capable of self-care, whereas 43 percent were found to be capable. When 50 of the 110 outcomes were individually investigated, only 5 percent of the subjects were probably not functioning at an optimal level.

The authors conclude that an additional 3 percent might have reached optimal functioning if existing follow-up procedures had been extended and made more routine. A lack of routine and regular follow-up was an important contributing factor in the loss of gains achieved in rehabilitation.

> ***Reviewers' Comments:*** This article may be of interest, but the study it reports is not experimental or quasi-experimental. It may be beneficial to occupational therapy personnel as an example of a quality assurance study.

**5** Andrews K, Brocklehurst JC, Richards B, Laycock PJ

CODES: P-2; T-2; S-1, 7, 19, 34, 40; M-1, 7, 8, 13, 14

# THE RATE OF RECOVERY FROM STROKE-- AND ITS MEASUREMENT

*International Rehabilitation Medicine* 3:155-161, 1981

A battery of tests was designed to measure improvement over time in the physical recovery of stroke patients and to compare the improvement with varying levels of disability at the onset of stroke. The study population consisted of 135 patients (71 males and 64 females) who had suffered an acute stroke and survived for at least two weeks. Thirty-four patients were under sixty-five years of age, 54 were between sixty-five and seventy-four years of age, and 47 were seventy-five years of age or older. Of this group, 94 were still alive at the end of the first year. Patients were examined at two weeks after stroke and subsequently at six-week intervals during the first year. The study was principally concerned with measurement of physical recovery. Muscle power, mobility, activities of daily living (ADL), walking, and independence were measured and coded with scoring and grading systems.

At onset 62 percent had shown moderate to severe impairment

of muscle power, and 88 percent had shown similar impairment in mobility and dependency. One year later 30 percent of the survivors remained dependent. Most patients had reached their peak levels of function within the first two months (71 percent for muscle power, 72 percent for ADL, and 88 percent for walking) except in the area of mobility (49 percent). The authors conclude that recovery from stroke extends over the first six months. Afterward, recovery is modest, much of it occurring in the severely impaired. The least recovery occurs in muscle power.

> *Reviewers' Comments:* This article is a worthwhile example of how to describe methods for use by others in their own research. Some good descriptive information is provided, and the conclusions are accurate based on the study as it is presented. The study focused on physical recovery. Other components, such as psychological factors and adjustment, were not addressed.

**6** Belcher SA, Clowers MR, Cabanayan AC

CODES:
P-2; T-7; S-1, 15, 19, 33, 39; M-1, 7, 8, 10, 11

# INDEPENDENT LIVING REHABILITATION NEEDS OF POSTDISCHARGE STROKE PERSONS: A PILOT STUDY

*Archives of Physical Medicine and Rehabilitation* 59:404-409, 1978

A pilot study was conducted to select dependent variables for a future independent living program for stroke patients. Seventy-three members of a stroke club in a large metropolitan area, and their spouses were interviewed in their homes at least one year after discharge from a hospital treatment program. The mean age of the population was sixty years. Forty-seven percent were males, and 53 percent were females. Fifty-eight percent were married, and 42 percent were single. Thirty-seven percent had suffered right cerebrovascular accidents (CVAs), 51 percent left CVAs, and 12 percent brain stem CVAs. The interview instruments included demographic data, the Barthel Index, the PULSES scale, the Social-Leisure Activity Scale, and the Service Identification Form.

Members of the sample stroke population perceived themselves as still having rehabilitation needs. Single and married people emphasized different needs, particularly in vocational rehabilitation. (The average monthly income for single stroke people was $369, for married people $1,120. That might explain the difference in this need.) The authors conclude that their findings indicate varying service needs, with implications for planning of rehabilitation programs.

> ### Reviewers' Comments:
> Design problems are evident, but the article provides some information about areas of rehabilitation for stroke patients. Occupational therapy personnel might consider focusing more attention on these, particularly in relation to the single person.

**7**  Belcher SA, Clowers MR, Cabanayan AC, Fordyce WE

CODES: P-2; T-7; S-1, 15, 33, 34, 39; M-1, 7, 10

## ACTIVITY PATTERNS OF MARRIED AND SINGLE INDIVIDUALS AFTER STROKE

*Archives of Physical Medicine and Rehabilitation* 63:308-312, 1982

An exploratory study was designed to look at social-leisure patterns and participation in commonplace activities among married and single individuals after stroke. People included had been discharged for at least one year from a medical treatment facility, were living in independent residences, and were not participating in a vocational rehabilitation program. The instrument used was the Activity Pattern Indicator (API), a behavioral frequency scale that is part of a set of instruments developed by the New York University Medical Center. The API was designed to measure how people spend their time. Subjects were forty-one married and thirty-two single stroke victims. Twenty-seven men and fifteen women were married and averaged sixty-two years of age; seven men and twenty-four women were single or living independently and had an average age of fifty-seven years.

Single people seemed to have reached a higher level of rehabilitation in that they received less assistance in personal care, did more household tasks, and had a more active level of social interaction. However, the data on married people did not discriminate between level of ability and need to perform. After stroke, married people showed less physical functioning and social interaction as measured by the API. This finding may not have indicated less real ability; rather, it may have reflected the presence of a spouse with whom to share tasks. Furthermore, the social activity data may have been influenced by age preference and level of income.

The authors acknowledge the small sample on which this study was based and conclude that the findings may not be representative of the total population. Also, there were restrictions in the matching of the two groups. As an exploratory study, it leaves many unanswered questions. However, it does introduce the use of behavioral technologies in evaluations and the measurement of social behavior as an indicator of rehabilitation status.

> *Reviewers' Comments:* The API is potentially useful, but there are a number of uncontrolled variables in the study. The study provides some tools that occupational therapy personnel could use in documenting the efficacy of services. The API seems to have promise for use in rehabilitation settings, and it is certainly consonant with an occupational behavior model of practice.

**8** Bell E, Jurek K, Wilson T

CODES:
P-2; T-7; S-1, 12,
21, 33, 40; M-1,
7, 8, 13, 14

# HAND SKILL MEASUREMENT: A GAUGE FOR TREATMENT

*American Journal of Occupational Therapy* 30:80-86, 1976

The Physical Capacities Evaluation (PCE), a measurement of hand skill was standardized by testing performance among an able-bodied population. The PCE comprised five unilateral hand skill tests, seven bilateral hand skill tests, and a dynamometer reading. The scores for each subtest were standardized by using a sample population of fifty subjects, thirty women and twenty men, aged nineteen to sixty-eight years. The test was then administered to patients with various types of disabilities: eighty paraplegics aged nineteen to fifty-seven years (twice as many men as women); forty-four right hemiplegics with a mean age of fifty years (equal numbers of men and women); and fifty left hemiplegics with a mean age of fifty-one years (equal numbers of men and women).

The performance of these patients and the implications for treatment are discussed. With paraplegic patients the test can be used to indicate a need for occupational therapists to develop hand skills suitable for employment requirements. With quadriplegic subjects the test may be useful to measure progress in developing skill in tenodesis function or to determine the potential value of functional orthosis. With hemiplegic subjects the test indicates the need for hand skill development of the uninvolved hand by measuring the skill of the functioning upper extremity.

Background information on the development of the PCE and a description of it are given. The authors conducted a follow-up study on thirty hemiplegic patients, measuring ability to dress. They report success in using scores on the PCE to determine readiness for dressing and propose that it be used to predict success in learning activities of daily living.

> *Reviewers' Comments:* This study provides another avenue for consideration in planning treatment programs. Assessments such as the PCE are greatly needed, and the
> ( continued on next page)

> PCE shows some promise.
> However, the design and the
> research as described are weak in
> terms of documentation, and there
> are flaws in the study's internal and
> external validity.

**9** Bourestom NC, Howard MT

CODES:
P-2; T-5; S-1, 12,
18, 34, 40; M-1,
7, 9

## BEHAVIORAL CORRELATES OF RECOVERY OF SELF-CARE IN HEMIPLEGIC PATIENTS

*Archives of Physical Medicine and Rehabilitation* 49:449-454, 1968

The validity of psychological tests in predicting the recovery of the self-care function in patients with hemiplegia resulting from cerebrovascular disease was explored. One hundred sixty subjects with hemiplegia were classified according to self-care status on admission to a rehabilitation program at the Kenny Rehabilitation Institute. Average admission occurred three months after onset. Subjects were sixteen to ninety-one years old with a mean age of sixty-four years. Left and right hemiplegia were almost equally represented. Patients were subclassified according to their degree of improvement during the rehabilitation program based on a 17-point, empirically derived self-care scale.

Psychological test scores covaried linearly with improvement in self-care. The discriminative powers of the tests varied according to the subjects' self-care status at the time of the initial psychological examination. For patients whose self-care activities were initially quite low, the performance IQ of the Wechsler Adult Intelligence Scale provided the best single measure for predicting the recovery of function in self-care. For patients requiring moderate or minimal assistance in self-care, the Porteus Maze Test and Part B of the Trail Making Test gave the most accurate prognosis. The authors conclude that the results clarify the relationship between psychological tests and self-care, reveal differences in the discriminatory powers of such tests, and can enable a more accurate prognosis of self-care recovery.

> **Reviewers' Comments:**
> Although this study is not recent, the material is of current value. However, those considering practical applications of these psychological tests in identifying the self-care potential of stroke patients should obtain further details from the authors.

**10**  Brocklehurst JC, Andrews K, Richards B, Laycock PJ

CODES:
P-2; T-5; S-1, 6,
19, 34, 40; M-1,
7, 8, 13, 14

# HOW MUCH PHYSICAL THERAPY FOR PATIENTS WITH STROKE?

*British Medical Journal* 279:1307-1310, 1978

The factors that determine type of physiotherapy and the extent to which the amount of treatment relates to the severity of stroke were explored in Great Britain. The study involved 135 patients who had suffered a stroke and survived for at least two weeks. Of the patients, 72 (53 percent) were male and 34 (25 percent) were under sixty-five years of age. Eighty-six (64 percent) of the patients were admitted to a general or geriatric hospital during the first two weeks after the onset of stroke. The remainder were admitted to a hospital beyond two weeks after stroke but before the end of the study period of one year. One hundred seven patients received physiotherapy, 35 received occupational therapy, and 19 received speech therapy. Occupational therapy was given for a more limited period than was physiotherapy, probably reflecting the limited availability of therapists. Those who received the most physiotherapy were the most severely involved and had the worst prognosis. Almost no recovery occurred after six months. Stiff and painful shoulders were present in 21 of the patients after two weeks and had developed in an additional 37 after one year.

The authors found that the amount of treatment given clearly related to the severity of the disability rather than to the potential for improvement. They conclude that the objectives of physiotherapy for patients with stroke need careful definition, with emphasis on treatment in the early months. They also suggest the need for appraisal of viable alternative types of care for the longer-term treatment of stroke patients whose disability is great and whose recovery is poor. This study does not afford a comparison of the effects of physical treatment on progress and recovery from stroke in matching treated and control groups, nor does it permit an assessment of the value of occupational therapy to patients with strokes.

> **Reviewers' Comments:**
> Although this study may not be generalizable to the United States, it does present some potential issues for further study by occupational therapists: (a) the effects of occupational therapy using this design model and (b) the need to assess the appropriateness and the length of treatment based on projected benefits.

## 11  Bryant NH, Candland L, Loewenstein R

CODES:
P-2; T-3; S-1, 10,
19, 22, 34, 39;
M-2, 7, 19, 20

# COMPARISON OF CARE AND COST OUTCOMES FOR STROKE PATIENTS WITH AND WITHOUT HOME CARE

*Stroke* 5:54-59, 1974

A study was undertaken to compare care and cost outcomes on two groups of stroke patients over a nine-month period. A first group of twenty-five patients received home care services. A second group of twenty-five patients received physical therapy services while hospitalized but did not receive home care services. Twenty-three of the twenty-five patients in the home care group were sixty-five years of age or over, and there were twelve males and thirteen females. The second group was matched by age and sex. Patients who had had extremely mild or severe strokes were eliminated from the study. Cost data and hospital days were not calculated until the patient was judged to be medically stable.

The hospital services used most frequently were physical therapy and social services. Occupational therapy, the intensive care unit, speech therapy, and inhalation therapy were used infrequently. Home care patients were found to have shorter hospitalizations, fewer readmissions for recurring stroke, fewer deaths, and lower overall costs. They tended to receive continuity of care, and could be discharged to themselves or their family and remain self-sufficient in the community.

> ***Reviewers' Comments:*** The study provides a model that supports the efficacy of home care services for stroke patients. However, it is primarily oriented toward the provision of physical therapy services. In addition, because the study took place in 1971, the cost data provided are outdated.

**12** Charait SE

CODES:
P-2; T-3; S-1, 6, 21, 22, 38; M-1, 8, 11, 14, 17

# A COMPARISON OF VOLAR AND DORSAL SPLINTING OF THE HEMIPLEGIC HAND

*American Journal of Occupational Therapy* 22:319-321, 1968

Twenty hemiplegic patients with spasticity of the affected hand were fitted with either volar or dorsal splints. The patients ranged in age from thirty to eighty years. There were ten men and ten women, nine with right hemiplegia and eleven with left. Splints were applied from four days to six years after the cerebrovascular accidents. Four patients had previously worn commercially made aluminum cock-up splints, and three had worn first volar, then dorsal splints. All patients were treated while in the hospital by physical therapists with passive- or active-range-of-motion exercises on an average of thirty minutes daily, five days a week. Several were treated with graded resistive exercise as well. None were treated with neuromuscular facilitation techniques. Splints were worn from two months to three years, two hours to twenty-three hours a day (removed only during bathing and physical therapy treatments). Spasticity was evaluated by an orthopedic surgeon, private physicians, and therapists.

The author found that the pressure of the volar splint on the palm of the hand appeared to facilitate the flexor muscles and in some cases to increase spasticity. The pressure of the dorsal splint on the back of the hand appeared to facilitate the extensors and reduce spasticity in their antagonists. Furthermore, maintaining the muscles in a position of prolonged stretch aided through inhibition. A dorsal splint might enhance this outcome. The constant wearing of splints had an adverse effect. Wearing splints only at night allowed more exercise and reduced stiffening of the joints during the day. The addition of neuromuscular facilitation techniques to reinforce the positive effects of the dorsal splint seemed indicated by the data but was beyond the scope of the study.

> ***Reviewers' Comments:*** The study is well presented, has historical value to the field, and supports the use of splints with this patient population. The author describes the splint designs and the materials used, but these have been replaced by newer materials and techniques.

**13** Chaudhuri G

CODES:
P-5; T-9; S-1, 19;
M-6, 13, 14, 16

# REHABILITATION OF THE STROKE PATIENT

*Geriatrics* 35:45-46, 49-50, 54; 1980

This article is an opinion statement and presents a general overview of various principles and issues surrounding stroke rehabilitation. The underlying premise is that stroke rehabilitation is effective and that the cost-effectiveness ratio of stroke rehabilitation is significant enough to offer therapy to every stroke victim. The effectiveness of stroke rehabilitation can be maximized and the costs minimized by following certain principles outlined by the author. The rehabilitation of the cerebrovascular accident patient is considered in three phases: the acute phase, the convalescent phase, and the delayed phase when complications are present. In the acute phase proper positioning is needed to prevent joint contractures. Rehabilitation through a team approach should begin as soon as the patient is medically stable and specific components of rehabilitation are delineated. Referral to a regional rehabilitation center or a specialized hospital unit is suggested. Here an individual assessment should be made, and a goal-oriented program designed. Discharge planning is discussed. It should include patient and family education and referrals to outpatient services or home care as necessary.

*Reviewers' Comments:* Much of this article is based on personal experience, and there is a lack of documentation to support the statements presented. However, the author does discuss several issues that are relevant for occupational therapy practice. First, therapy and rehabilitation are important after hospitalization, and occupational therapists should ensure that they occur. They include trial home visits and home health services, occupational therapy included. Second, treatment must be reassessed periodically. Third, the role of family members is important in the rehabilitation process.

**14** Chin PL

CODES:
P-4; T-11; S-1,
22; M-5, 8, 14

## PHYSICAL TECHNIQUES IN STROKE REHABILITATION

*Journal of the Royal College of Physicians of London* 16:165-169, 1982

This educational review advocates the use of a continuum of rehabilitation activities directed toward the maintenance of optimum function. A rationale for a variety of physical therapy treatment approaches is discussed based on a review of the literature. Physical rehabilitation of stroke patients uses manual techniques for restoration of function, including conventional and facilitation exercises and the application of physical agents and equipment. Physical agents, such as heat, light, sound, water, and electricity, are used for management of painful shoulders and relief of muscle spasm. There is sufficient clinical evidence to warrant selective use of these agents with hemiplegic patients in accordance with demonstrable patient preference. The aim of therapeutic exercises is to restore function; the dilemma is whether to optimize residual function or to maximize recovery from disability. Optimization is a pragmatic approach to the restoration of self-care by using special equipment, training the unaffected side, and preventing contractures. Alternatively, to retrain hemiplegic limbs to function as normally as possible, the use of facilitation and inhibition regimens is favored. These movement therapy techniques are based on the premise that posture and sensory stimuli can modify abnormal reflex patterns that emerge after cerebral damage.

A survey of techniques has shown that a combination of conventional, functionally oriented exercises and facilitation exercises is most popular, particularly proprioceptive neuromuscular facilitation and Bobath techniques. Because these techniques consume large amounts of physiotherapy time, research regarding their efficacy is warranted. However, evaluation is difficult because there is a lack of standardization in measurement and a failure to discriminate between benefit and effectiveness.

Several studies with controlled trials of exercise regimens are summarized, although the findings do not yield decisive guidelines.  The author proposes a phased task-oriented approach in the application of physical therapy techniques to the stroke patient.

> ***Reviewers' Comments:***  This article offers some viable suggestions regarding the application of triage principles in determining which patients could benefit most from treatment and cost-effective ways to allocate resources.  The author defines disability and emphasizes that it is the "difference between what the patient can do and what is actually done at home."  The article's relevance to occupational therapy rests with the reader's ability to generalize to the areas of practice that overlap those of physical therapy.

**15**  Coughlan AK,  Humphrey M

CODES:
P-2; T-2; S-1,
12, 19, 33, 40;
M-3, 7, 8, 9, 10

## PRESENILE STROKE:  LONG-TERM OUTCOME FOR PATIENTS AND THEIR FAMILIES

*Rheumatology and Rehabilitation* 21:115-122, 1982

Long-term outcomes for stroke patients with right hemiplegia, left hemiplegia, or no hemiplegia were compared in England. Questionnaires were mailed to the spouses of 395 surviving patients who had attended a medical rehabilitation center three to eight years earlier and met the following criteria:  under age 65 at the time of stroke, married at the time of attendance at the rehabilitation center, and known not to have been incapacitated by ill health before the stroke.  A total of 170 questionnaires were returned, yielding a 43-percent response rate.  Included in the analysis were 103 men and 67 women, with a mean age at the time of stroke of 51.6 years. The survey requested information on mobility, self-care, communication, work, health, and enjoyment of life.

Problems of self-care were reported as persisting in about two-thirds of the patients. Restricted mobility was reported in one-half. Only one-third of those who were working at the time of their stroke and were still below retirement age at follow-up were employed. Memory problems, marked personality changes, and language disorders affected more than one-third. Approximately one-third reported marked loss of enjoyment of life. Treatment services for depression or tension were sought by one-third of the patients and their families. Few differences in outcome for left and right hemiplegics were noted. The authors suggest that many patients, particularly those with severe hemiplegia, and their spouses would benefit from counseling services.

> *Reviewers' Comments:* This is thorough and soundly done research. It provides beneficial information about long-term outcomes. The consideration of depression and of the need for community services is of particular interest.

**16** Denes G, Semenza C, Stoppa E, Lis A

CODES:
P-2; T-3; S-1, 11,
22, 34, 39; M-1,
7, 8, 13, 14

## UNILATERAL SPATIAL NEGLECT AND RECOVERY FROM HEMIPLEGIA: A FOLLOW-UP STUDY

*Brain* 105:543-552, 1982

This follow-up study sought to prove the existence of interhemispheric differences in recovery patterns and to measure their effect on cognitive, attentional, and emotional disturbances as well as on motor skills. The investigation was undertaken in the department of physical therapy of a hospital in Padova, Italy, in 1975-1976. After exclusion of an initial ninety patients, the study population consisted of two groups of twenty-four patients matched in age, sex, schooling, interval between onset and therapy, and amount of physical therapy, differentiated only by side of lesion. After six months, left hemiplegics showed poorer outcomes functionally and socially, as had been generally observed. Unilateral spatial neglect, more frequent and more severe in the left hemiplegics, seemed to be crucial in hampering their performance. The explanation offered for this is that the right parietal lobe can be activated by visual stimuli projected onto either field and therefore seems to be able to compensate for a left hemisphere lesion; the reverse is not possible.

The authors note that their data are at variance with earlier studies showing the side of lesion not to be a significant factor in the process of recovery. However, those studies measured recovery by muscle strength or function, and motor recovery does not ensure functional improvements in stroke patients. The present study stresses the importance of functional improvement to social adjustment; the importance of a neuropsychological approach to studying changes following brain damage; and the probable importance of such assessment in therapeutic approaches designed to overcome a patient's disabilities.

> *Reviewers' Comments:* The study is well designed and complete. Occupational therapists need to consider the conclusions related to functional improvement and their role in the recovery process.

**17**  Diller L, Buxbaum J, Chiotelis S

CODES:
P-2; T-5; S-1,
12, 19, 34, 40;
M-1, 7, 8, 9, 10, 13

# RELEARNING MOTOR SKILLS IN HEMIPLEGIA: ERROR ANALYSIS

*Genetic Psychology Monographs* 85:249-286, 1972

Five factors related to learning a functional motor skill were investigated: the differential effects of the side of hemiplegia; the effects of organicity; the relationship between the extent of therapist assistance and patient styles of behavior; sensorimotor and psychological correlates of levels of assistance and errors in learning; and interrelationships among factors. The study involved sixty-three right hemiplegics (thirty-four males and twenty-nine females, with a mean age of 61.7 years) and fifty-six left hemiplegics (thirty-six males and twenty females, with a mean age of 62.6 years) undergoing inpatient treatment in a rehabilitation program. Patients had all suffered cerebrovascular accidents as adults, and their need for training in activities of daily living (ADL) was the critical point for being considered suitable for the study.

No significant differences in demographics for right and left hemiplegic groups were found. Levels of assistance and errors were similar in right and left hemiplegics, indicating that the side of hemiplegia was unrelated to competence. However, these measures related to different variables for right than for left hemiplegics, suggesting that different factors entered into the mastery of a functional skill for the two groups. Errors appeared to have different functional relationships in the two groups. No differences were found in terms of the extent of organicity.

The best measures for predicting outcome in level of assistance were reported as initial level and a clinical rating of "organicity." Progress in ADL appeared to occur in "slow steps." When a change in therapist occurred, patients evidenced setbacks in levels of assistance. The most organic patients showed the greatest number of setbacks.

> *Reviewers' Comments:* The study is well done and contains considerable information. It supports the use of ADL measures for baseline data. The discussion of differences between groups is useful. The comments about the effects of a change in therapist are of interest.

**18**  Feibel JH, Springer CJ

CODES:
P-2; T-5; S-1, 15,
34, 39; M-1, 7, 8,
9, 10

## DEPRESSION AND FAILURE TO RESUME SOCIAL ACTIVITIES AFTER STROKE

*Archives of Physical Medicine and Rehabilitation* 63:276-278, 1982

A community-wide cohort of stroke patients was followed to determine the incidence of depression and the characteristics of depression-prone patients. The study also looked at the relationship of depression to the patient's level of dependence or independence in activities of daily living (ADL), mobility, and extent of resumption of premorbid social activities. A total of ninety-one stroke patients, with a mean age of 72.2 years, was selected for study between May and July 1977. The patients were identified through a telephone network established with seven acute care hospitals in Monroe County, New York. Each patient's diagnosis was verified, and the patients completed ten-day, two-month, and six-month poststroke assessments. The patients were assessed by trained, registered nurses. The assessments included demographic and clinical features as well as disposition status. Physical independence in ADL and mobility were determined using the Katz scales. Depression status was determined by nurses' observations. Somatic complaints and information about patients' participation in social activities both before and after stroke were also obtained.

The incidence of depression was 26 percent ($N$ = 24) six months after stroke. Depression was significantly correlated with failure to resume premorbid social activities. Depressed patients showed a reduction of 67 percent of their prior social activities, whereas nondepressed patients lost a mean of 43 percent of their prior social activities ($p$ < 0.01). Depression status was not significantly related to age, sex, marital or cognitive status, or the side of brain involvement. Independence in ADL and ambulation and change in residence after stroke also were not significantly related to depression status. The authors conclude that because depression is common after stroke, is associated with failure to return to previous activities, and cannot be predicted by commonly used patient characteristics, the health care team must carefully identify, monitor, and manage depression in the patient recovering from stroke.

> ***Reviewers' Comments:*** The research design, including the small sample and the interrater reliability, is questionable. However, the article points out the importance of psychosocial adjustment factors. It would be interesting to study failure to return to previous activities and depression after other medical conditions. Occupational therapists might consider replicating this study.

**19** Feigenson JS

CODES:
P-5; T-9; S-1, 12, 19, 41; M-5, 19

## STROKE REHABILITATION: EFFECTIVENESS, BENEFITS, AND COST. SOME PRACTICAL CONSIDERATIONS (EDITORIAL)

*Stroke* 10:1-4, 1979

This editorial reviews current data on the effectiveness, benefits, and costs of stroke rehabilitation. Information is presented to help physicians select the most cost-effective treatment for patients suffering from a cerebrovascular insult.

Among the findings and guidelines are these:
• Patients with multiple diagnoses do not have a longer length of stay in disability-oriented rehabilitation than in acute care. Therefore, treatment and duration of hospitalization should be based on functional and neurological deficits rather than on diagnostic category.
• Early intervention decreases the length of stay and increases functional return. Therefore, rehabilitation in the acute care

hospital should begin as soon as a patient is medically stable.
• Specialized stroke care units do not incur additional costs.
Therefore, rapid referral to disability-oriented regional
rehabilitation facilities should be initiated, if such facilities are
available.

Although the article does not identify other health care
providers by profession, occupational therapy services are
implied. A suggested method for improving benefits to the
patient is to emphasize how a patient spends a typical day. Areas
for research are proposed that compare measures of patient
satisfaction with premorbid and postmorbid life-styles.

> *Reviewers' Comments:* This
> article supports many of the current
> practices of occupational therapy,
> such as educating physicians,
> community, and family about the
> value of early intervention;
> emphasizing interdisciplinary
> collaboration for the total care of
> the stroke patient; and
> incorporating family members and
> friends as extenders of
> rehabilitation services. In
> considering outcomes, concern for
> the quality of a patient's life is as
> important as increasing function.

**20** Feigenson JS

CODES:
P-3; T-11; S-1, 7,
12, 16, 19; M-5,
7, 13, 19

## STROKE REHABILITATION: OUTCOME STUDIES AND GUIDELINES FOR ALTERNATIVE LEVELS OF CARE

*Stroke* 12:372-375, 1981

This review refers to various background articles related to
outcomes of stroke care and proposes that failure to provide
rehabilitation services for patients with persistent stroke deficits

may in the long run be more costly than providing them. A stratified health care delivery system that offers alternative levels of care may benefit the patient, his or her family, and society at the lowest possible cost. Stroke units offering acute and rehabilitative care in hospitals have proved cost-effective, as have regional rehabilitation facilities and skilled nursing/chronic care homes. After discharge, many patients still have severe residual deficits requiring multidisciplinary care and regular medical supervision. These services can be provided in alternative settings, including home care, day-care programs, day hospital programs, limited outpatient treatment, and stroke clubs. Each of these is briefly described in terms of type, duration, intensity, and reimbursement for services.

The author concludes that stroke rehabilitation could "salvage" up to 80 percent of the patients who are now referred to nursing homes for poststroke care, and that rehabilitation is an effective way of treating physical disabilities. The available information suggests that rehabilitation is cost-effective and that early intervention can significantly decrease morbidity and mortality while improving functional outcome. By providing comprehensive care from the onset of stroke through long-term follow-up, physicians can maintain their patients at the highest possible functional level yet hold down the high cost of long-term institutional care.

> *Reviewers' Comments:* More data to substantiate the author's bias toward rehabilitation would make the article persuasive for use with nonrehabilitation personnel.

**21** Feigenson JS, Gitlow HS, Greenberg SD

CODES:
P-2; T-3; S-1, 12, 19, 34, 40; M-1, 7, 8, 13, 14, 19

# THE DISABILITY ORIENTED REHABILITATION UNIT--A MAJOR FACTOR INFLUENCING STROKE OUTCOME

*Stroke* 10:5-8, 1979

Data on 667 patients admitted to the Burke Rehabilitation Center were abstracted and prospectively studied from the Center's stroke data base. Patients formed two groups, 589 admitted to the disability-oriented stroke unit (SU) and 78 admitted to other units at the center (NSU). Demographic characteristics, staffing patterns, and therapeutic programs were similar.

In general, SU patients were weaker on admission, had longer intervals between the onset of stroke and admission, and exhibited more concurrent medical problems and neurological deficits than NSU patients. Nevertheless, at discharge SU patients went home more often and ambulated at a higher level than NSU patients did. There were no significant differences between SU and NSU patients in activities-of-daily-living status and length of stay. Despite their greater impairment SU patients made more progress in the same length of time than NSU patients. Costs for SU and NSU patients were essentially similar. No additional costs were incurred by the hospital in changing to disability-oriented patient care, because the staff-patient ratio was not altered.

Possible explanations given for the improved outcomes include improved communication within the multidisciplinary team, a more consistent approach to problem solving, increased staff interest and expertise through specialization, and better patient interaction within a homogeneous group. The authors conclude that even in a specialized rehabilitation center a disability-oriented approach to stroke care can significantly improve outcome without increasing costs to the patient or the facility.

*Reviewers' Comments:* This is a well-written study. Details of the intervention program are reported to be provided in other articles. The study supports the use of stroke units. The details of the cost analysis referred to by the authors are not given.

# 22 Feigenson JS, McCarthy ML

CODES:
P-6; T-7; S-1, 12,
19, 34, 40; M-13,
14, 16

## STROKE REHABILITATION, PART 2: GUIDELINES FOR ESTABLISHING A STROKE REHABILITATION UNIT

*New York State Journal of Medicine*, Aug 1977, pp 1430-1434

Findings reported in part 1 of this series (see abstract no. 24) are summarized, and possible factors responsible for the high success rate in returning patients to their home are discussed. Information is provided on the types of program activities that are important to reinforce the interdisciplinary team concept. The distinct responsibilities of each team member, including the occupational therapist, are described, as well as this program's expectation that each professional participate in all stroke unit activities. The staff were trained to promote continuity of care, open communication, and a questioning approach to problem solving. Beneficial features of the rehabilitation center's program that are described include the admission procedure, the daily routine, family/patient education, and discharge planning.

Based on follow-up data over thirty-three months, 80 percent of 566 stroke patients were discharged to home after forty-five days in the rehabilitation unit. Furthermore, 85 percent were ambulatory and 54 percent needed no assistance with activities of daily living. A literature review of comparable studies indicated that this outcome was unusually high. Other stroke rehabilitation units are encouraged to examine the guidelines offered, as a way of improving outcomes by altering program emphasis without making major organizational or budgetary changes.

*Reviewers' Comments:*
Together, parts 1 and 2 provide a well-written and informative set of materials on outcomes and the team approach. The authors reinforce the concept of multidisciplinary/ interdisciplinary collaboration as central to the treatment of chronic

(continued on next page)

and/or debilitating illnesses, such as stroke. Further, they provide information on the types of activities that are important to reinforce a team concept. For those who have never worked with a team of providers, the articles provide sufficient incentive to seek out a rehabilitation team, observe its programming, and consider implementing a similar approach.

## 23

Feigenson JS, McCarthy ML,
Greenberg SD, Feigenson WD

CODES:
P-2; T-3; S-1, 12,
19, 34, 40; M-1,
7, 8, 9

# FACTORS INFLUENCING OUTCOME AND LENGTH OF STAY IN A STROKE REHABILITATION UNIT, PART 2: COMPARISON OF 318 SCREENED AND 248 UNSCREENED PATIENTS

*Stroke* 8:657-662, 1977

The outcome and the length of stay for a control group of 248 unscreened patients and a group of 318 patients medically and socially screened before admission, were compared. (Findings related to the control group are reported in part 1 of the article abstracted here--see abstract no. 25). All patients were discharged from the same thirty-bed stroke unit over a period of thirty-three months. The average age of the screened patients was sixty-seven years; the range was seventeen to ninety. There were 145 males and 173 females and approximately equal numbers with right and left hemiparesis. Diagnostic categories, the age distribution of males and females, and the age distribution of patients with right and left hemiparesis were essentially similar to those of the controls. Data on 312 patients (98 percent of the original 318) were appropriate for analysis. Outcome was defined in terms of discharge disposition, ability to perform activities of daily living (ADL), ability to walk, and length of stay.

Preadmission medical, neurological, and social service screening did not improve the overall outcome or reduce the length of stay. A program aimed at identifying and treating perceptual and cognitive dysfunction did improve functional status and discharge disposition in patients having perceptual, but not cognitive, deficits. A detailed analysis of the factors influencing outcome and length of stay confirmed and extended earlier findings:

1. Severe weakness on admission and long intervals between the onset of stroke and admission were adversely related to outcome, as were perceptual or cognitive dysfunction, poor motivation, a homonymous hemianopsia, multiple neurological deficits, and poor functional status on discharge.
2. Dysphasia, a hemisensory loss, age (under eighty years), and concurrent arteriosclerotic heart disease, hypertension, or diabetes were unrelated to outcome.

It was demonstrated that most patients, even those with unfavorable prognostic signs, significantly improved after appropriate treatment programs. Factors influencing outcome and length of stay are listed.

*Reviewers' Comments:* This is a clear, well-conceived study that follows up on the authors' previous research and builds on earlier findings. Although the article was published in 1977, it is still germane to the field, and the results are pertinent for occupational therapy personnel. It would have been beneficial to include more information on the screening procedures used as admission criteria Nonetheless, as in part 1, the authors point out the salience of specific clinical problems to the rehabilitation of the stroke victim. The article should prove useful to occupational therapists in determining which patients can be most helped by intervention.

# 24

Feigenson JS, McCarthy ML,
Meese PD, Feigenson WD,
Greenberg SD, Rubin E, McDowell FH

CODES:
P-2; T-4; S-1, 12,
19, 34, 40;
M-2, 7, 8

## STROKE REHABILITATION, PART 1: FACTORS PREDICTING OUTCOME AND LENGTH OF STAY--AN OVERVIEW

*New York State Journal of Medicine,* Aug 1977, pp 1426-1430

Predictors of outcome defining groups that might receive maximum benefit from rehabilitation were analyzed. The study cohort was a group of 566 elderly stroke patients treated in a short-term stroke rehabilitation unit at Burke Rehabilitation Center over a period of thirty-three months. The patients comprised 269 males and 297 females who had been discharged from the stroke rehabilitation unit. The distribution of left and right hemiparesis was nearly equal. The average age was sixty-seven years; the range was seventeen to ninety-eight. Descriptive data were abstracted from a computerized stroke discharge summary. Outcome was defined in terms of discharge disposition, activities-of-daily-living status, and ambulation status.

Severe weakness, perceptual or cognitive dysfunction, homonymous hemianopsia or multiple neurological deficits, poor motivation, inability to walk, and persistent urinary/fecal incontinence were clearly identified as poor prognostic indicators. A hemisensory loss, dysphasia, the age of the patient, and concurrent arteriosclerotic heart disease, hypertension, or diabetes were unrelated to outcomes. Outcome statistics link neurological deficits to functional deficits and the length of stay. The statistics reported help define a group of stroke patients who may benefit maximally from rehabilitation. They also outline factors that may increase the length of stay. Finally, they underscore the fact that most stroke patients make significant gains in a suitable rehabilitation program even if they have one or more signs of a poor prognosis.

> ***Reviewers' Comments:***
> Comments are reported under abstract no. 22, which summarizes part 2 of the article abstracted here.

**25** Feigenson JS, McDowell FH,
Meese P, McCarthy ML,
Greenberg SD

CODES:
P-2; T-3; S-1, 12,
19, 34, 40; M-1,
7, 8, 9, 19

# FACTORS INFLUENCING OUTCOME AND LENGTH OF STAY IN A STROKE REHABILITATION UNIT, PART 1: ANALYSIS OF 248 UNSCREENED PATIENTS--MEDICAL AND FUNCTIONAL PROGNOSTIC INDICATORS

*Stroke* 8:651-656, 1977

A retrospective analysis was conducted of 248 patients with stroke (average age sixty-seven years, range seventeen to ninety-eight) admitted to a stroke rehabilitation unit over a sixteen-month period. Patients participated in three or four sessions of occupational, physical, or speech therapy per day and received activities-of-daily-living (ADL) training from nursing staff and aides. Length of stay, ADL, and discharge disposition data were abstracted from a computerized discharge summary.

Results showed that 80 percent of the patients were able to return home after an average length of stay of forty-three days. At discharge 85 percent of the group were ambulatory, and 56 percent required no help in ADL. Severity of weakness on admission, long intervals between the onset of stroke and admission, and severe perceptual or cognitive dysfunction or a homonymous hemianopsia in addition to a motor deficit were related to an unfavorable outcome and an increased length of stay. The age of the patient, dysphasia, or a hemisensory deficit in addition to weakness, diabetes, hypertension, and arteriosclerotic heart disease were unrelated to the patient's functional status on discharge, discharge disposition, or length of stay. Many patients with unfavorable prognostic signs made significant improvement after admission and were subsequently discharged. Although the findings may facilitate prediction of which patients can make maximal gains in a short-term treatment facility, they also show that most patients, even those with "poor prognostic signs," can make enough functional improvement to be managed at home after a relatively short hospitalization.

> *Reviewers' Comments:* This article presents sufficient documentation and has an acceptable research design. It provides current and important information for occupational therapy personnel and other members of rehabilitative teams concerned with patient/client factors and clinical problems that may influence outcomes.

**26** Feldman DJ, Lee PR, Unterecker J, Lloyd K, Rusk HA, Toole A

CODES:
P-2; T-3; S-1, 6, 19, 34, 39; M-1, 7, 8, 9

## A COMPARISON OF FUNCTIONALLY ORIENTED MEDICAL CARE AND FORMAL REHABILITATION IN THE MANAGEMENT OF PATIENTS WITH HEMIPLEGIA DUE TO CEREBROVASCULAR DISEASE

*Journal of Chronic Disease* 15:297-310, 1962

The results of functionally oriented medical care and a formal rehabilitation program for a group of patients with physical or neuromuscular deficit secondary to cerebrovascular disease were compared in a randomized, controlled study. Eighty-two patients met established conditions for inclusion in the study and were randomly assigned to either a control group ($N = 40$) receiving functionally oriented medical care or an experimental group ($N = 42$) receiving formal rehabilitation services. The majority of the patients were over sixty years old. Fifty males and thirty-two females were studied. The patients were classified in terms of neuromuscular deficits and functional status in activities of daily living. The degree of intellectual impairment was also assessed.

The final evaluation revealed that 12 percent of the rehabilitation group and 27.5 percent of the control group had little or no physical impairment at the termination of the program. The rehabilitation group demonstrated more achievement in level

of function and greater levels of function for each level of
physical impairment.

> ***Reviewers' Comments:*** The
> study's statistical validity is
> debatable because of the small
> number in the categorized groups.
> Descriptions of the differences
> between the rehabilitative program
> and the functional medical care
> program are limited. The study
> raises questions regarding which
> patients will benefit most from
> rehabilitation and considers the
> possibility of negative effects of
> formal rehabilitation on physical
> function.

**27**  Forer SK, Miller LS

CODES:
P-2; T-3; S-1, 12,
19, 34, 40;
M-1, 7, 9

# REHABILITATION OUTCOME: COMPARATIVE ANALYSIS OF DIFFERENT PATIENT TYPES

*Archives of Physical Medicine and Rehabilitation* 61:359-365,
1980

A study was conducted to provide comparative follow-up data
on patients in the Comprehensive Medical Rehabilitation Unit of
the Rehabilitation Institute in Glendale, California, and their
progress in the community at one year to nineteen months after
discharge. A comparative analysis of various patient types was
conducted on postdischarge progress with regard to eating,
dressing, transfers, bladder management, ambulation, cognition,
language comprehension and speech, placement, and mortality
rates. The population consisted of 263 patients differentiated by
diagnostic group. Their rehabilitation stay averaged 23.7 days,
after which 77 percent were discharged to private homes and the

remaining 23 percent were placed in more restrictive environments. Patients' functional levels of competency in activities of daily living (ADL) and cognitive activities were rated at admission and at discharge using a modified Hospital Utilization Project (HUP) program. The HUP patient data system, developed in response to needs identified by the Comprehensive Medical Rehabilitation Unit, provided a systematic mechanism for reporting various outcomes at the time of discharge and comparing them with admission status and follow-up. In October 1978, twelve to nineteen months after discharge, follow-up data were obtained by structured telephone interviews on the progress of the 192 patients still alive.

The majority had continued to improve in functional competency in ADL and in cognitive areas after discharge. Some showed statistically significant gains. The prognosis for continued functional improvement appeared excellent for cancer and cerebrovascular accident (CVA) patients, fair to good for brain-stem-infarction and general debility patients, limited for amputee and head trauma victims, negligible for patients with arthritic and spinal cord injuries, and poor for patients with neurological conditions and back or neck pain. On cognitive items CVA patients with right hemiparesis made the most progress, although they were the most impaired at discharge. An extremely high correlation was found between the patients' satisfaction with their present level of adjustment and their satisfaction with inpatient services. The authors conclude that longitudinal evaluations by diagnostic group may determine which types of patients can benefit most from a comprehensive medical rehabilitation unit. Further studies should compare treatment program designs and control for spontaneous recovery.

*Reviewers' Comments:* The conditions studied include those treated by occupational therapy personnel, although occupational therapy and the other therapies are not specifically mentioned. The information could be useful to those making decisions about deploying resources. An occupational therapist was probably part of the team based on progress having been measured in
(continued on next page)

areas of ADL customarily managed by occupational therapy personnel. However, contact with the authors would be necessary to confirm this. Some of the significant findings may be due to the large number of subjects or the large number of statistical tests conducted.

# 28

Garraway WM, Akhtar AJ,
Hockey L, Prescott RJ

CODES:
P-2; T-3; S-1, 7,
19, 34, 40; M-3,
7, 10

## MANAGEMENT OF ACUTE STROKE IN THE ELDERLY: FOLLOW-UP OF A CONTROLLED TRIAL

*British Medical Journal* 281:827-829, 1980

Follow-up data are provided on a group of elderly stroke patients who were studied in a randomized controlled trial that is reported in an earlier article by the same authors (see abstract no. 29). In the original study, patients were assigned to either a stroke rehabilitation unit or general medical units. The follow-up was undertaken to establish whether gains made during hospital treatment were maintained after discharge. All 192 patients available for follow-up (101 from the stroke unit and 91 from the medical unit) were visited monthly, and an index of nursing dependency was administered. This index was designed to establish the degree of assistance the patients received when performing activities of daily living during the twenty-four hours preceding each visit. The follow-up period lasted for one year. At the end of the trial, functional outcome was reassessed using hospital discharge criteria.

Patients with acute stroke treated in the stroke unit were returned to independence at the time of discharge in a larger proportion than those treated in medical units. However, the gains made during hospitalization were not maintained over the long term. Only 55 percent of the stroke unit patients (56) were reassessed as independent, and 19 percent (13 of 67 previously independent patients) had regressed to dependency. In contrast, 57 percent of the medical unit patients (52) remained independent, and 24 percent (11 of 45 previously dependent patients) had progressed to independence.

Factors that might have contributed to these changes are identified. It is suggested that stroke unit patients regressed because of overprotection by their families, who were made aware of the patients' disabilities by stroke unit staff but were not informed of the need to maintain the gains made during acute rehabilitation. Thus, during the follow-up year independent patients from the stroke unit were allowed to do less than independent patients from medical units, and dependent patients from medical units were allowed to do more than their counterparts from the stroke unit. Furthermore, because of overcrowding on medical units, those patients were discharged sooner, perhaps before they had attained their full potential. Consequently the natural course of their improvement continued at home.

The authors conclude that although the results do not negate the worth of stroke units, they do confirm that management of stroke continues well beyond the acute phase and requires the cooperation of all concerned with the patient. The findings suggest the importance of patient and family education in the rehabilitation process.

> *Reviewers' Comments:* The study confirms that management of stroke continues well beyond the acute hospital phase. As the authors note, the data do not provide conclusive evidence as to why the improvement advantage realized by stroke patients at the time of discharge was not found at one-year follow-up. However, the possible explanations offered deserve consideration by occupational therapy personnel.

# 29

Garraway WM, Akhtar AJ,
Prescott RJ, Hockey L

CODES:
P-2; T-3; S-1, 7,
21, 22, 24, 34, 40;
M-1, 7, 13, 14, 17

## MANAGEMENT OF ACUTE STROKE IN THE ELDERLY: PRELIMINARY RESULTS OF A CONTROLLED TRIAL

*British Medical Journal* 280:1040-1043, 1980

A randomized controlled trial conducted from October 1975 to April 1978 compared the management of patients admitted to a stroke unit ($N = 155$) with that of patients admitted to medical units ($N = 152$). The mean age was seventy-three years. On selection for the study the two groups had no significant differences in age, sex, social class, marital status, home situation, activities before stroke, and duration of stroke. The use of physiotherapy, occupational therapy, and speech therapy was also assessed. The outcome of the acute phase of rehabilitation was measured using an activities-of-daily-living assessment when discharge was imminent or at sixteen weeks after admission.

A significantly higher proportion of the patients discharged from the stroke unit (78 of 155, or 50 percent) were assessed as independent, compared with the patients discharged from medical units (49 of 152, or 32 percent). Eighty-eight percent of the patients admitted to the stroke unit received occupational therapy, compared with 47 percent of the medical unit patients. Two-thirds of all patients in the stroke unit had begun occupational therapy within one week after admission, compared with 18 percent of the medical unit patients. No great differences were found for speech therapy. The proportion of patients receiving physiotherapy was higher in the stroke unit group than in the medical unit group, and stroke unit patients began physiotherapy services earlier than the medical unit group did. The authors conclude that establishing a stroke unit improves the natural history of stroke by increasing the proportion of patients who return to functional independence.

NOTE: An Efficacy Data Brief on this article is available from the American Occupational Therapy Association, Quality Assurance Division.

> *Reviewers' Comments:* The study contributes evidence to support the role of occupational therapy in a stroke rehabilitation unit and suggests the efficacy of early intervention.

## 30 Garraway WM, Akhtar AJ, Smith DL, Smith ME

CODES:
P-2; T-3; S-1, 11, 19, 34, 40; M-1, 7, 8, 13, 17

# THE TRIAGE OF STROKE REHABILITATION

*Journal of Epidemiology and Community Health* 35:39-44, 1981

Triage was used to select geriatric stroke patients for a randomized controlled trial of the effectiveness of rehabilitation. The study was designed to test the hypothesis that the proportion of patients who could be returned to independence would be higher for those admitted to a stroke unit than for those admitted to medical units. The authors proposed that a system of triage similar in concept to that used by military surgeons would enable the identification and the selection of acute stroke patients who were most likely to benefit from rehabilitation. Patients sixty years of age or older were classified into one of three bands-- lower, middle, or upper--based on their initial stroke presentation (e.g., their degree of consciousness, the presence of hemiplegia, and their skill in activities of daily living) and their prognosis. The middle-band patients, who were described as conscious at the onset of stroke, were selected for the study. Concentrating on the middle band allowed a more realistic comparison of the relative effectiveness of a stroke unit and medical units in rehabilitating patients whose prognosis in terms of years of life was good but who were likely to have a residual disability that would require ongoing support.

A total of 584 patients were visited at home by a medical staff member of the research team to confirm the diagnosis of stroke made by a general practitioner and to determine eligibility for the study. A total of 311 patients were placed in the middle band and admitted to either a stroke unit or a general medical unit through a system of restricted randomization. The authors conclude that a stroke unit can return a higher proportion of patients to independence than medical units can.

Data on stroke patients who were not included in the randomized trial are discussed. An analysis of the triage criteria, estimates of the incidence of strokes, and projections of the bed capacity of stroke units are also provided.

*Reviewers' Comments:* The article does not provide information specific to occupational therapy practice or management, because the occupational therapy aspect of the rehabilitation effort is not defined. However, occupational therapy appears to have been employed in the rehabilitation process if one judges by the criteria used to assess functional independence and the outcome of the acute phase of rehabilitation. The article may be of benefit in terms of its consideration of the rehabilitation effort in general.

**31**  Garraway WM, Walton MS, Akhtar AJ, Prescott RJ

CODES:
P-2; T-3; S-1, 11, 19, 34, 40; M-1, 7, 10, 13, 16

# THE USE OF HEALTH AND SOCIAL SERVICES IN THE MANAGEMENT OF STROKE IN THE COMMUNITY: RESULTS FROM A CONTROLLED TRIAL

*Age and Ageing* 10:95-104, 1981

Follow-up data were collected on elderly stroke patients who were studied during a randomized controlled trial that compared the management of patients on a stroke unit with that of patients on medical units. The original study has been reported in the literature (see abstract no. 29). Follow-up data were gathered for one year, dating from the time patients were discharged or sixteen weeks after admission. A total of 125 stroke unit patients and 109 medical unit patients entered follow-up. All patients were visited at monthly intervals, and an index of nursing dependency was administered to determine the level of assistance that the patients received in the performance of activities of daily living. The use of hospital services (including outpatient clinics, day hospitals, occupational therapy, physiotherapy, and speech therapy) and the use of community services (including general practitioners, health visitors, community nurses, social workers, home help, chiropodists, Meals on Wheels, and voluntary agencies) were recorded.

Patients from the stroke unit received more health and social services than patients from medical units did, particularly in the initial follow-up period. The use of services was not related to functional outcome of patients at hospital discharge. No overall differences were found between the groups.

The authors determine that no clear conclusions can be drawn from the use of health and social services in the long-term management of patients who participated in the controlled trial. However, they offer possible explanations of the findings. They also discuss the limitations of the study, attributable to the lack of criteria for measuring the *actual need* for services, which may differ from the *use* of services, and the lack of criteria for providing services.

> *Reviewers' Comments:* The study reinforces the importance of specific criteria for admission, discharge, and determination of functional independence. The article is well written and sound from a research point of view.

**32**  Gordon EE, Kohn KH

CODES:
P-2; T-3; S-1, 6,
12, 19, 34, 39;
M-1, 7, 8, 9, 10

# EVALUATION OF REHABILITATION METHODS IN THE HEMIPLEGIC PATIENT

*Journal of Chronic Disease* 19:3-16, 1966

An investigation was conducted to compare the achievement of hemiplegic patients who received full-scale rehabilitation services at a rehabilitation center, with patients who received restorative services from a rehabilitation nurse in a general hospital. One hundred eighty-one potential subjects were considered for the study. Ninety were rejected for several reasons, including a lack of potential for improvement due to intellectual deterioration or severe physical impairment; a lack of need for physical rehabilitation; acute medical or surgical conditions; and neurological deficits too severe for the rehabilitation resources of a general hospital and a nurse. Patients with aphasia were also excluded. Fifty-six patients (thirty-eight females and eighteen males) with an average age of 64.4 years were assigned to the group who received services at the rehabilitation center. Thirty-five patients (twenty-two females and thirteen males) with an average age of 64.9 years were assigned to the general hospital and the services of a rehabilitation nurse. The two groups were similar on a number of patient parameters.

Differences in locomotion and cognitive flexibility (as measured by the Shure-Wepman test) were noted. Self-care and improvements in living arrangements were equally affected by the rehabilitation team and the rehabilitation nurse. Patients in the group that received full-scale rehabilitation services demonstrated greater improvements in locomotion than the other group did. The authors conclude that severely involved individuals require the services of a rehabilitation center. It is difficult to generalize the findings because of differences between the study population and the typical general hospital population.

> *Reviewers' Comments:* The research is not current, and the article's contributions to occupational therapy practice are limited. Research questions are not clearly defined, and caution must be exercised in interpreting the experimental conditions and the role of the rehabilitation nurse.

# 33 Granger CV, Sherwood CC, Greer DS

CODES:
P-2; T-5; S-1, 6, 7, 10, 19, 34, 40; M-1, 7, 8, 9, 10

## FUNCTIONAL STATUS MEASURES IN A COMPREHENSIVE STROKE CARE PROGRAM

*Archives of Physical Medicine and Rehabilitation* 58:555-561, 1977

A study was conducted of 269 patients who were followed for approximately two years through a coordinated care system consisting of a hospital acute stroke unit, a rehabilitation unit, and community care in Fall River, Massachusetts. Functional status data were recorded on long-range evaluation summaries, and assessments were conducted on admission and discharge from hospital units and at six months after discharge. Adaptations of the Barthel Index and the PULSES Profile were used for self-care and mobility assessments. The total study population comprised 136 men and 133 women, with a mean age of 70 years.

From the acute care unit 48 percent returned home, 16 percent were transferred to a rehabilitation unit, 20 percent were discharged to long-term care, and 16 percent died. Patients transferred to the rehabilitation unit were more impaired than those discharged to home but less impaired than those transferred to long-term-care facilities. A rehabilitation subgroup of 45, 26 men and 29 women, with a mean age of 69.8 years, was analyzed. Forty-seven percent were discharged to the community. Correlation and discriminant function analyses were performed to display relationships between clinical measures and outcomes. Outcomes in terms of type of discharge were heavily dependent on gaining a level of independence that corresponded to a score of 61 or better on the Barthel Index. A strong correlation with discharge scores on the Barthel Index and the PULSES Profile and clinical outcome assignments (e.g., discharge to home versus transfer to a rehabilitation unit) was noted. A Barthel score of 21 or better at the time of admission for acute stroke and 41 or better at the time of transfer for rehabilitation favored a discharge to home with a score of 61 or better (within nine weeks of the onset of stroke).

> *Reviewers' Comments:* The authors are very brief in their descriptions of how they conducted the study, so it is difficult to evaluate the quality of the research. The article includes some important ideas on prognosis, outcomes, and the efficient use of rehabilitation services.

**34** Greenberg S, Fowler RS Jr

CODES:
P-2; T-3; S-1, 16, 21, 34, 39; M-1, 8, 14

# KINESTHETIC BIOFEEDBACK: A TREATMENT MODALITY FOR ELBOW RANGE OF MOTION IN HEMIPLEGIA

*American Journal of Occupational Therapy* 34:738-743, 1980

The effectiveness of kinesthetic biofeedback in the treatment of hemiplegia was assessed in an experiment using twenty patients with limited elbow extension secondary to a cerebrovascular accident (CVA). Patients were randomly assigned to one of two treatment groups: a control group, with which an occupational therapy approach aimed at increasing functional use of the involved upper extremity was used; and an experimental group, to which audiovisual kinesthetic feedback was given. The procedure for providing the feedback was as follows: An electrogoniometer was attached to the lateral aspect of the affected arm with the fulcrum at the elbow joint. When a specificied amount of extension was attained, a green light was activated and a tone increased in pitch. The ten subjects were treated twice a week for four weeks in half-hour sessions. The control group was treated with therapeutic techniques derived from the Brunnstrom approach.

The results indicated that kinesthetic biofeedback was of equal therapeutic value to, but no more effective than, conventional therapy. The data suggested that age, sex, and the length of time beyond one year after the CVA did not affect outcomes. Aphasic subjects benefitted equally. A majority of subjects improved on variables not directly related to treatment, such as increased motivation, heightened body awareness, and a determination to improve self-care skills. Several subjects assumed an active role and might have been capable of working independently with the biofeedback equipment in a clinical setting. The equipment would be able to furnish some of the motivation and the reinforcement usually provided by a therapist and, if used independently, would decrease the cost of one-to-one treatment sessions. Hemiplegia patients can continue to improve over time. The authors conclude that the use of biofeedback techniques in outpatient settings may make long-term treatment of the chronically disabled financially feasible.

*Reviewers' Comments:* This article highlights the beneficial use of kinesthetic biofeedback as a reinforcement and a motivating technique in occupational therapy that allows the patient to work independently. Also of interest are the results showing that one year after a CVA, this particular patient population continued to benefit from a rehabilitation program, whether through a conventional approach or the use of kinesthetic biofeedback.

# 35 Gresham GE

CODES:
P-5; T-7; S-1, 6,
14, 19, 34, 36;
M-5, 7, 8, 13, 14, 17

## REHABILITATION OF THE GERIATRIC PATIENT: STROKE REHABILITATION, THE REHABILITATION TEAM, AND THE USEFULNESS OF FUNCTIONAL ASSESSMENT

*Primary Care* 9:239-247, 1982

The author's opinion is presented on the importance of incorporating the principles and the techniques of rehabilitation medicine in the care of the older person. The multidisciplinary approach of rehabilitation is particularly important with the geriatric patient, for whom functional preservation must be considered simultaneously with functional enhancement and restoration. Salient features of rehabilitation in the elderly are illustrated through the case history of a stroke patient. Some disability may be the result of a concurrent disease process that may require management and a modification of the rehabilitation program. Motor strength, perceptual integrity, and the ability to learn are prime factors in the successful rehabilitation of a stroke survivor. Advanced age should not be a deterrent to a trial of rehabilitation, but its complications must be considered. Elderly patients may progress too slowly for placement in intensive hospital-based rehabilitation units; consideration of alternative settings and levels of care is a critical factor.

The concept of functional preservation is particularly relevant to geriatric medicine. Once optimum functional enhancement has been achieved, the geriatric patient must be kept at that level as long as possible, and comprehensive care should include programs and services oriented toward this goal. Periodic functional evaluation should be done to detect any possible decline in functional status, and early intervention of rehabilitation services should be considered as a preventive measure. It is suggested that this be done through the use of a standardized functional assessment instrument such as the Barthel Index. This approach can provide valuable information for program monitoring, utilization review, justification for third-party payers, exchange of information between institutions, and data for statistical analysis.

*Reviewers' Comments:* This article provides general information and is of value mainly for its recommendation of standardized functional assessment and its support of the Barthel Index. The author underscores the need for careful planning to place the patient in the most appropriate setting.

# 36   Harasymiw SJ, Albrecht GL

CODES:
P-2; T-7; S-1, 12,
19, 40; M-2, 7,
19, 20

## ADMISSION AND DISCHARGE INDICATORS AS AIDS IN OPTIMIZING COMPREHENSIVE REHABILITATION SERVICES

*Scandinavian Journal of Rehabilitative Medicine* 11:123-128, 1979

To optimize admission and discharge decisions, a model correlating the components of time, costs, use of services, and functional levels was tested. Rehabilitation progress and outcome were conceptualized in terms of functional gains from treatment. The model assessed the dollar costs of increasing the level of function by one unit as measured by the Barthel Index. (Cost/function indicators can be used to assess whether a patient or a diagnostic group is ready to benefit from intensive rehabilitative services. For example, patients with low functional ability may not be strong enough for rigorous treatment and should remain in acute care facilities. Likewise, patients with high Barthel scores have less room for improvement and may progress as well in less cost-intensive environments.) The model was tested with data from a random sample of medical records, including those of 97 spinal cord injury and 132 focal cerebral patients, the majority of whom suffered hemiplegia as a result of stroke. Data were drawn from ten leading comprehensive rehabilitation centers in the United States.

The model's basic structure was supported by the data. Its use as an aid in managing patients, evaluating services, planning new programs, and developing computer-simulated models of the cost effectiveness of rehabilitation is recommended.

> *Reviewers' Comments:* This study may be more relevant to management than to clinicians in its approach to cost effectiveness and the development of theoretical models. It supports the concept that there may be a way of determining who is most likely to benefit from therapy and in what setting. It reiterates the importance of timeliness in treatment and emphasizes that there are optimum times for rehabilitation services to occur in the recovery process of stroke and spinal cord injury patients.

# 37 Harrison H

CODES:
P-2; T-2; S-1, 10,
21, 34, 36; M-1,
7, 8, 17

## THE ROLE OF THE PRESSURE SPLINT IN SENSORY STIMULATION OF THE HEMIPLEGIC UPPER EXTREMITY

*North Carolina Occupational Therapy Association Selected Papers,* Oct 1982, pp 8-14

An occupational therapist reviews the literature on sensory receptors and their relationship to motor function. The clinical use of the pressure splint in the treatment of sensory deficits in hemiplegia is featured. A case study of a seventy-one-year-old male with a diagnosis of vertebral-basilar disease and resultant right hemiparesis and left hypesthesia is presented. A pressure splint was applied to each upper extremity for fifteen minutes two to three times per week for a total of thirteen sessions. The pressure splint was the only prescribed treatment modality used for all sessions. The results of sensory and functional status testing were compared with initial evaluation findings. Improvements in sensory and functional status were noted.

> **Reviewers' Comments:**
> Replication is necessary because this is a single case study. The documentation is not sufficient for validation analysis. Major flaws threaten the study's internal and external validity. However, the study does present helpful information on neuroanatomy and neurophysiological theory, and a bibliography of related readings for the practitioner is included.

**38** Honer J, Mohr T, Roth R

CODES:
P-2; T-2; S-1, 16, 22, 34, 36; M-1, 8, 10, 14

# ELECTROMYOGRAPHIC BIOFEEDBACK TO DISSOCIATE AN UPPER EXTREMITY SYNERGY PATTERN: A CASE REPORT

*Physical Therapy* 62:299-303, 1982

The effectiveness of electromyographic (EMG) biofeedback training in disrupting the synergistic patterns of the upper extremity in a hemiplegic patient was evaluated. The patient was a sixty-six-year-old male who had suffered a right cerebrovascular accident eleven months before the study. The patient's level of function in the left upper extremity was assessed before, midway through, and after biofeedback training. A passive-range-of-motion test was also administered. The goal of treatment was deviation from a flexor synergy pattern by training increased contraction of the anterior deltoid muscle with accompanying elbow extension. A Cyborg BL-933 with auditory and visual components and the capacity to monitor two muscle groups simultaneously was used. Each session contained fourteen contraction-relaxation sequences. Twenty-two sessions were conducted on successive weekdays. The Likert scale, a self-reporting instrument, was administered after each session and included questions on ability to concentrate, degree of fatigue, and happy, sad, and anxious feelings.

Active range of motion through the flexor synergy remained essentially unchanged, and no deviations from the synergies were obtained. Passive range of motion did not improve from the pretraining level. Considerable variability in EMG values was noted. A significant positive correlation was found between concentration and contraction. Increased anxiety and increased concentration were also significantly related. Greater anxiety was associated with increased contraction of the anterior deltoid. The authors conclude that the presence of marked spasticity in antagonist muscle groups may preclude successful EMG biofeedback training.

> *Reviewers' Comments:* The study supports the use of biofeedback in a specific case and gives impetus to further investigations to compare this approach with that of functional activity. Major flaws threaten the study's external and internal validity, however.

**39** Hurd MM, Farrell KH, Waylonis GW

CODES:
P-2; T-3; S-1, 6, 19, 38; M-1, 8, 11, 17

# SHOULDER SLING FOR HEMIPLEGIA: FRIEND OR FOE ?

*Archives of Physical Medicine and Rehabilitation* 55:519-522, 1974

Fourteen acute hemiplegic patients were studied to determine whether the commonly used hemisling applied to the flail upper extremity of the acute hemiparetic patient is a clinically helpful or harmful device. For nine months the fourteen patients meeting the study criteria were assigned to an experimental (sling applied) or a control (no sling) group. In all other respects, patients were treated identically. The patients underwent detailed initial and follow-up examinations, including neurological testing; evaluation of joint range of motion of the involved upper extremity; and electromyographic evaluation of both upper extremities, the involved lower extremity, and the paracervical muscles. The complete evaluation was repeated two to three weeks later and again at three to seven months after the cerebrovascular accident (CVA). Nine patients were observed for three months or longer. Areas of major concern were shoulder range of motion, shoulder pain, glenohumeral subluxation, and possible peripheral nerve injury. The authors also hoped to determine if there was a relationship between the use of the sling and the posthemiplegic reflex sympathetic dystrophy syndrome.

The results indicated no appreciable difference in shoulder range of motion, shoulder pain, or subluxation. Further, no evidence of an increased incidence of peripheral nerve injury or plexus injury was apparent in the patients treated without a sling. The authors conclude that there is no evidence to suggest that the hemisling be uniformly applied or considered essential in the care of the flail upper extremity after a CVA. However, the shoulder sling may be of value to assist in ambulation.

*Reviewers' Comments:* The study raises important issues in assessing the therapeutic value of a common practice, that is, the use of the upper extremity sling with post-CVA patients. The sample is small and follow-up data are sparse. Thus, the external validity of the study suffers.

**40**   Inaba M, Edberg E, Montgomery J,
Gillis MK

CODES:
P-2; T-3; S-1, 12,
22, 33, 39; M-1,
7, 8, 13, 14

# EFFECTIVENESS OF FUNCTIONAL TRAINING, ACTIVE EXERCISE, AND RESISTIVE EXERCISE FOR PATIENTS WITH HEMIPLEGIA

*Physical Therapy* 53:28-35, 1973

The effectiveness of programs of progressive resistive exercise, simple active exercise, and training in activities of daily living (ADL) in attaining functional independence in hemiplegia patients was compared. Patients admitted to a rehabilitation unit who met the following criteria were included: a cerebrovascular accident (CVA) secondary to thrombosis, embolus, or intracerebral hemorrhage; an ability to follow directions; sufficient strength in the affected lower limb to push a specified weight; and an inability to walk independently. A physical therapist who was not involved in the treatment program evaluated the patients. The patients were randomly assigned to one of three treatment groups. Group I, the control group (twenty-six patients with a mean age of 56.88 years), received only functional training and selective stretching. Group II (twenty-three patients with a mean age of 56.11 years) received active exercise in addition to the control group program. Group III (twenty-eight patients with a mean age of 55.89 years) received progressive resistive exercise in addition to the control group program. The groups differed minimally in etiology of the CVA, sex, side of hemiplegia, age, activities of daily living, and extension strength.

More patients in Group III made significant improvements in ADL and demonstrated more gains in strength after one month of treatment than patients in Groups I and II did, but no significant differences were noted after two months of treatment. The authors conclude that the most effective one-month treatment for achieving functional independence for the population under study is a program consisting of selective stretching, training in ADL, and progressive resistive exercise. Progressive resistive exercise is more effective in improving strength than programs of ADL alone or ADL combined with active exercise.

> *Reviewers' Comments:*
> Although the article does not give
> specific information on the
> therapists or the amount of
> treatment received, it appears to
> describe a good basic study.

# 41 Isaacs B

CODES:
P-4; T-7; S-1, 11,
19, 34, 40; M-1,
7, 8, 13, 16

## FIVE YEARS' EXPERIENCE OF
## A STROKE UNIT

*Health Bulletin* 35:94-98, 1979

This article, an educational review, gives an account of a thirty-bed stroke unit established at Lightburn Hospital, Glasgow, Scotland, and provides some results of its operation from 1969 through 1973. A total of 715 patients were admitted to this stroke ward in the five years under review. They were a severely disabled group with a high prevalence of disorders of communication and perception, and they were not representative of all stroke patients or even of all hospitalized stroke patients. Despite these factors, outcomes were encouraging. Of the 587 stroke patients treated soon after onset, 53 percent were discharged to home, 26 percent were transferred for long-term inpatient care, and 22 percent died. Of those discharged to home, nearly two-thirds had left the hospital within two months.

Follow-up studies revealed that the level of physical independence was maintained after discharge. Patients who went home to live alone did better than those who went to live with a spouse or relatives. The latter group suffered social and psychological distress. Their problems resulted in the formation of three stroke clubs: one for former patients, one for families, and one for those coping with dysphasia. All of these groups met at the hospital. Other successful innovations included discussion groups for patients, the use of diaries to enhance communication with staff, and a daily activities program in the ward. The rehabilitation team included occupational therapists.

The authors conclude that the stroke unit formed a focus of major clinical interest and demonstrated the value of multidisciplinary collaboration. It allowed for a more comprehensive assessment of all aspects of the patient's illness and disability, it enhanced awareness of the objectives of rehabilitation for staff and family, and it played a valuable educational role.

> *Reviewers' Comments:* The article offers some programming ideas that, although generated ten years ago, maintain some relevance today. It also provides a potential area of follow-up and collaborative study for occupational therapists and social workers concerning postrehabilitation adjustment for those who live alone and those who live with others. However, the phenomenon reported warrants further validation.

**42** Isaacs B, Marks R

CODES:
P-2; T-5; S-1, 11,
19, 34, 39; M-1,
7, 8, 9, 13, 14

# DETERMINANTS OF OUTCOME OF STROKE REHABILITATION

*Age and Ageing* 2:139-149, 1973

The outcomes of a stroke rehabilitation program in which patients received physical therapy, occupational therapy, or speech therapy were studied. An attempt was also made to classify patients by type of disorder into four clinical groups and to relate clinical features to outcome data. The four groups were right hemiplegia with a significant communication disorder (twenty-seven cases), right hemiplegia with no significant communication disorder (nineteen cases), left hemiplegia with a significant perceptual disorder (twenty-one cases), and left hemiplegia with no significant perceptual disorder (twenty cases). The study group comprised one hundred patients admitted consecutively to the stroke ward at Lightburn Hospital in Glasgow, Scotland, from September 1970 to May 1971. Thirteen patients were excluded, leaving a sample of eighty-seven (forty-six males and forty-one females). Twenty-five were under age sixty-five, thirty-nine were aged sixty-five to seventy-four, and twenty-three were aged seventy-five and over.

Forty-eight patients were discharged to home, nineteen were transferred to continuing care wards, and twenty died while in the hospital. The factors associated with a favorable outcome were age under sixty-five years and the absence of severe cognitive disturbance. Satisfactory results were obtained in alert patients with disturbances of perception or communication, or with accompanying heart disease. The differences in outcome data for the four clinical groups were small. The authors conclude that simple tests of cognitive and perceptual function should be a part of the clinical examination of stroke patients accepted for rehabilitation, and they support the use of such tests as guides to management and treatment planning.

> *Reviewers' Comments:* This study is of value in its support of (a) cognitive testing for assessing potential outcomes, (b) the role of cognitive functioning in gaining functional independence, and (c) cognitive retraining. However, the documentation is not sufficient for a full validation analysis.

**43** Jain S

CODES:
P-2; T-2; S-1, 12, 19, 33, 36; M-1, 7, 10, 13, 14, 16

# OPERANT CONDITIONING FOR MANAGEMENT OF A NONCOMPLIANT REHABILITATION CASE AFTER STROKE

*Archives of Physical Medicine and Rehabilitation* 63:374-376, 1982

An operant learning approach was evaluated by a multidisciplinary team of therapists at the Rehabilitation Institute of Chicago. The subject was a fifty-three-year-old former schoolteacher with a diagnosis of left hemiplegia secondary to stroke. She was a difficult rehabilitation patient. In the hospital she was depressed, was noncompliant in learning activities of daily living (ADL), refused to eat, and, except for physical therapy, frequently missed or was unmotivated in therapy sessions. A unified program was designed to teach her new appropriate behaviors and reduce the incidence of inappropriate behaviors. Her husband and all of the therapists presented a similar system of rewards and coordinated and supported one another's activities. Good performances in ADL were rewarded with small privileges, increased eating was rewarded with extra physical therapy, and attendance and good performance in therapies were rewarded with weekend passes.

Immediately after initiation of the program there was a dramatic increase in appropriate behaviors. A three-month follow-up reevaluation indicated that the patient was actively involved in volunteer work and no longer depressed. Her husband substantiated her gains, which were maintained at one year. The author concludes that the study supports a further expansion and application of operant conditioning research in rehabilitation.

> *Reviewers' Comments:* The article's references and examples may be of interest to those new to behavioral approaches. The study is valid from a research perspective.

**44** Kaplan J, Hier DB

CODES:
P-2; T-5; S-1, 12, 34, 39; M-1, 7, 8, 9

# VISUOSPATIAL DEFICITS AFTER RIGHT HEMISPHERE STROKE

*American Journal of Occupational Therapy* 36:314-321, 1982

The influence of visuospatial deficits on functional status after a right hemisphere stroke was investigated in thirty-four patients. Seventeen men and seventeen women ranging from 47 to 79 years of age (with a mean of 66.9 years) were studied. Patients were consecutively drawn from admissions to a neurological unit in a rehabilitation hospital over a six-month period. Criteria for selection included age below 80 years, no previous history of stroke, right-handedness, and orientation as to person, time, and place. A control group of eight men and eight women of comparable age and education who were hospitalized for nonneurological conditions was also tested. Patients were examined for the degree of hemiparesis, hemianopia, and tactile extinction, and received psychological tests. Their level of independence in self-care was assessed at admission, every two weeks during hospitalization, and at discharge.

Little correlation was found between the severity of hemiparesis and the severity of visuospatial deficits. However, both motor and visuospatial deficits were important predictors of functional status at the time of discharge. Discharge disposition status, discharge self-care score, and changes in self-care scores were influenced by visuospatial deficits. Hemiparesis, verbal ability, educational level, and the interval between the onset of illness and admission to the rehabilitation unit did not correlate with visuospatial deficits. Visuospatial ability declined with age. The authors conclude that visuospatial deficits are an important independent factor governing functional outcome and should be given as much attention as hemiparesis during discharge and rehabilitation planning for patients with a right hemisphere stroke.

*Reviewers' Comments:* The research is current and may provide some useful information on visuospatial deficits of patients with right hemisphere stroke.

**45** Kinsella G, Ford B

CODES:
P-2; T-5; S-1, 12, 18, 34, 39; M-1, 7, 8, 9

# ACUTE RECOVERY PATTERNS IN STROKE PATIENTS: NEUROPSYCHOLOGICAL FACTORS

*Medical Journal of Australia* 2:663-666, 1980

Acute functional recovery after stroke was evaluated in thirty-one moderately disabled patients to discern patterns in rehabilitation as a function of time. The subjects comprised seventeen with left hemisphere damage and fourteen with right hemisphere damage. The mean age was sixty-two years. There was no significant difference between the hemisphere groups in sex or age. The study sought to explain early recovery patterns in this group of stroke patients and to evaluate various ideas about unilateral spatial neglect. Assessments were made at intervals of four, eight, and twelve weeks. The Northwick Park Activities of Daily Living Index and various measures of mobility level were used, as well as a neuropsychological battery that assessed unilateral spatial neglect, constructional apraxia, right-left orientation, planning skills, ideomotor apraxia, aphasia, and the ability to memorize and learn new tasks. Assessments were selected to identify and measure the areas that contributed to outcome in functional terms, not to provide comprehensive analyses of behavioral deficits. The influence of the site of the insult on recovery was also evaluated.

When the time variable was applied to changes in functional abilities and intellectual competence, different patterns emerged. Significant recovery in functional abilities occurred between the four- and eight-week assessments, with improvement tapering off to insignificant by the twelfth week. No significant improvement in intellectual/cognitive abilities was noted over time.

No hemispheric difference in recovery rate was found unless the patient also demonstrated unilateral spatial neglect as part of the deficit syndrome. Unilateral spatial neglect was exclusively found in patients with right hemisphere lesions and emerged as a factor associated with poor outcome. Subjects with unilateral spatial neglect remained impaired at twelve weeks on complex tasks that did not rely on mobility alone, implying that this intellectual deficit is a potent source of disability for which new methods of remediation are needed.

These results have implications for the timing and the intensity of the delivery of active rehabilitation therapy. They also raise questions about the adequacy of rehabilitation programs designed to remediate unilateral spatial neglect.

*Reviewers' Comments:* The contributions of this study include suggestions that intervention should occur early for maximum usefulness, that a need exists for better retraining techniques for

(continued on next page)

cognitive and perceptual skills, that recovery may not be related to hemisphere specialization, and that cognitive-perceptual factors such as unilateral spatial neglect may be significant in the recovery of activities of daily living.

**46**  Labi MLC, Phillips TF, Gresham GE

CODES:
P-2; T-3; S-1, 12, 19, 34, 40; M-1, 3, 7, 10

## PSYCHOSOCIAL DISABILITY IN PHYSICALLY RESTORED LONG-TERM STROKE SURVIVORS

*Archives of Physical Medicine and Rehabilitation* 61:561-565, 1980

Three parameters of social function--socialization in the home, socialization outside the home, and hobbies and interests--were analyzed to determine the social reintegration of long-term survivors with documented completed strokes. Data were drawn from the work of the Framingham study group (1972-1975), described in other literature. A total of 121 survivors (56 men and 65 women) and 141 controls met the initial criteria of having a minimum score of 20 on the Kenny Self-Care Evaluation, indicating satisfactory levels of physical function.

The findings revealed that many stroke survivors did not return to a normal social life even after physical disability had ceased to be a serious obstacle. Comparisons between the survivor and control groups were statistically significant on all three parameters of social functioning. Greater difficulty was shown in resuming activities outside the home than inside the home. Better-educated persons tended to function less well socially than did those with less education, and women had a greater decrease in interests and hobbies than men did. Much of this social disability could not be accounted for by age, physical impairment, or specific neurological deficit. The documented distribution of functional disabilities suggested that psychosocial factors, as well as organic deficits, were major determinants. The authors conclude that rehabilitation programs need to help patients and families anticipate and cope with the psychosocial problems resulting from stroke, thereby reducing the risk of social isolation.

*Reviewers' Comments:* In general, this is a well-done study and a well-written article that demonstrates the need for psychosocial rehabilitation for stroke patients. Some data and information about the study are not included, and some conclusions in the discussion section are not supported with evidence of statistical significance.

# 47

Lehmann JF, DeLateur BJ,
Fowler RS Jr, Warren CG, Arnhold R,
Schertzer G, Hurka R, Whitmore JJ,
Masock AJ, Chambers KH

CODES:
P-2; T-5; S-1,
12, 19, 33, 40;
M-1, 7, 8, 19

## STROKE: DOES REHABILITATION AFFECT OUTCOME?

*Archives of Physical Medicine and Rehabilitation* 56:375-382, 1975

A sample of 114 stroke patients admitted to a rehabilitation center was studied statistically to measure functional gains achieved and retained after therapy. Levels of independence were evaluated by correlating each patient's functional gains with the level of independence he or she obtained after treatment. To measure function, a functional profile was developed that evaluated seven activities, each according to a 5-point scale. The sample distinguished between patients admitted more than six and more than twelve months after stroke, to control for spontaneous recovery.

Significant gains were recorded and retained by both groups that could not be attributed merely to spontaneous recovery. Some independence was lost in self-feeding skills. The influence of rehabilitation gains in determining the ultimate living arrangement of patients after discharge was assessed. All had lived independently (alone, with family, or with a spouse) at the onset of stroke. Seventy-three percent returned to living independently after discharge, and at follow-up 75 percent had achieved this level of independence. Those who returned to nursing homes did so at a higher functional level and therefore needed a lower and consequently less costly level of care. The results of an estimated cost-benefit ratio were encouraging. Using 51.2 months as an average poststroke survival time, the authors determined the break-even point in rehabilitating patients who returned home to be 21.5 months. For those who required nursing home care, it was 35.2 months. This cost-benefit analysis showed that intensive stroke rehabilitation paid for itself by improving the disposition of patients. The authors conclude that expenditures for rehabilitation therapy result in significant financial savings for society and significant independence for patients.

NOTE: An Efficacy Data Brief on this article is available from the American Occupational Therapy Association, Quality Assurance Division.

*Reviewers' Comments:* This is important evidence for cost-benefit validations. Although the research is not current, studies such as this are seldom reported. Thus, it is a valuable piece of work. It supports the long-term benefits of rehabilitation (i.e., six to twelve months after onset), provides cost-benefit data attesting to the value of rehabilitation, offers evidence of communities' needs for treatment facilities, and justifies the value of rehabilitation to referring individuals and/or agencies.

48 Lehmann JF, DeLateur BJ,
Fowler RS Jr, Warren CG, Arnhold R,
Schertzer G, Hurka R, Whitmore JJ,
Masock AJ, Chambers KH

CODES:
P-2; T-5; S-1, 12,
19, 34, 40; M-1,
7, 8, 9, 10

## STROKE REHABILITATION: OUTCOME AND PREDICTION

*Archives of Physical Medicine and Rehabilitation* 56:383-389, 1975

To ensure the most efficacious use of rehabilitation facilities and services, an attempt was made to compile a list of predictors of rehabilitative success. In this retrospective study of 114 stroke patients admitted consecutively to a tertiary care facility, patient charts were evaluated to discriminate between patients with good or poor rehabilitative prognoses and to determine if a modification of the therapeutic intervention might have altered the predicted outcome. The items assessed for predictive value were medical data, age, functional levels at admission and discharge, results of psychological tests, family support, income, and educational level. The same predictors were used to analyze final disposition of the patient at discharge.

Predictors of functional outcome that showed some correlation with successful rehabilitation were medical data, age, results of psychological tests, and educational level. None of these predictors showed a correlation with outcome high enough to allow precise prediction in individual cases. They did, however, provide general indicators for the patients with severe functional impairment who were more likely to gain from a rehabilitation program. The older patient with a more extensive and severe lesion, signs of congestive heart failure, generalized arteriosclerosis, gross perceptual deficit, and a lower level of education was identified as less likely to improve in a rehabilitation program. There was no correlation between the severity of functional impairment at admission and the gains obtained in the rehabilitation program.

The authors conclude that, overall, the identified predictors are not accurate enough to predict gains in the rehabilitation process or disposition of individual patients. Therefore, no one should be denied a therapeutic trial. In analyzing the relationship of the predictors to the final disposition of patients at discharge, it was found that family income and support were of value but medical data were not. Because family involvement can sometimes be changed by a therapeutic team, this predictor may also present a major target for intervention.

> *Reviewers' Comments:* This is part 2 of a study conducted by the same authors (see abstract no. 47). The sample and the type of rehabilitation care the patients received are described in the initial work. This study suffers from some methodological flaws in the types of measures and analytical approach used. However, it offers a worthwhile argument for family support as a reasonable target of treatment intervention. It also stresses the importance of a therapeutic rehabilitation trial for even the most severely involved patient because prediction of outcome on an individual basis is not possible.

**49** McCann BC, Culbertson RA

CODES:
P-2; T-3; S-1, 6, 19, 40; M-2, 7, 8, 10, 13, 14

# COMPARISON OF TWO SYSTEMS FOR STROKE REHABILITATION IN A GENERAL HOSPITAL

*Journal of the American Geriatrics Society* 24:211-216, 1976

A study was conducted at Rhode Island Hospital to determine the comparative effects of two stroke rehabilitation programs on the outcomes of treatment. The results of data on 224 patients in an eight-bed stroke unit were compared with those of 110 patients treated on the medical service of the same hospital. Patients were treated on the medical service only if they could not be accommodated on the stroke unit because its beds were all occupied. The stroke unit was designed as a therapeutic community to enhance patient morale and motivation. Outcomes were measured on a 4-point rating scale, with level 1 referring to mild disability and level 4 referring to profound disability.

Level-3 patients, those with severe disabilities that limited their ability to function except with supervision, significantly improved more on the stroke unit than on the medical service. Level-2 patients, those with moderate impairment requiring occasional assistance, did well in either setting. Level-4 patients did poorly in both. Occupational therapy was not reported as a part of the multidisciplinary approach, although the nursing staff role included measuring functional assessment, stimulating activities of daily living, and setting realistic goals for independence. More level-3 patients were treated in the stroke unit sample, making the two groups (stroke unit and medical service) nonequivalent on one of sixteen variables. The authors suggest that the difference in outcome for level-3 patients may be attributable to the organization of the stroke unit service: a greater number of physical therapy sessions, an increased length of hospital stay, family involvement, and specialized nursing care. The authors also suggest that one reason for the difference in numbers of level-3 patients between groups may have been selective referral by physicians, based on their perception of the unit's success with this population.

> *Reviewers' Comments:* The heuristic value of this study lies in its identification of a specific subgroup of a general disease category that may benefit most from a particular available resource. However, the study has major flaws in its internal and external validity based on the nonequivalence of the two groups and the fact that the results cannot be generalized.

**50** McClatchie G

CODES:
P-2; T-2; S-1, 12,
19, 34, 40; M-1,
7, 8, 13, 14

# SURVEY OF THE REHABILITATION OUTCOME OF STROKES

*Medical Journal of Australia* 1:649-651, 1980

The results of a prospective survey of 174 stroke patients treated in "a fast-stream approach" in a rehabilitation unit in Sydney, Australia, are described. Much of the data were supplied by members of the multidisciplinary team, including occupational therapists. Measures of outcome were tabulated in four areas: motor status, sensory deficits, functional status, and communication skills.

Marked improvement was noted in motor and functional status. The interactive effects of motor and sensory deficits were critical at all outcome levels. Balance was shown to be a more important discriminant for mobility than any parameter of motor function. Results of before and after measures of communication skills indicated modest improvement. Family support was identified as an important factor in disposition. In this sample 126 patients went home, 35 went to a nursing home, 2 went to a hostel, and 11 went to an acute care hospital. The length of stay was only loosely related to the severity of stroke. Medical complications and placement problems contributed to lengths of stay in excess of sixty days.

The author sought to provide outcome data as a justification for the intensive treatment of selected stroke patients. Further, the author attempted to demonstrate the need for social agencies to support the patient at home. The fast-stream approach is not clearly defined in the article. However, it is described in an unpublished study referenced by the author.

> ***Reviewers' Comments:*** Data collection categories, quantitative comparisons of outcomes, and discussion of the factors influencing disposition may be of interest and suggest researchable
> (continued on next page)

questions. Caution should be taken against generalizing results from a descriptive study.

**51** Moskowitz E, Lightbody FEH, Freitag NS

CODES:
P-2; T-7; S-1, 12, 19, 34, 40; M-3, 7, 8, 10, 11

## LONG-TERM FOLLOW-UP OF THE POSTSTROKE PATIENT

*Archives of Physical Medicine and Rehabilitation* 53:167-172, 1972

The medical history, the clinical assessment, and the functional status of 518 poststroke patients were assessed. Patients were enrolled in a hemiplegia registry for metropolitan New York that compiled data on the long-term complications and health needs of stroke survivors, using the PULSES Profile. Of the 518 patients, follow-up examinations were performed on 313 over a three-year period.

Data analysis disclosed numerous findings with implications for rehabilitation. Only 32 percent of the subjects were considered independent, in part due to a lack of orientation of the family during initial hospitalization and after discharge from a rehabilitation program. Return of function was not always consistent with motor recovery, which usually peaks within six months. During periodic reevaluations by the stroke team, functional changes in the PULSES Profile reflected deterioration, resulting from superimposed complications such as intercurrent illness, trauma, or contractures. A continued overuse of slings and a failure to repair braces also caused deterioration. In these cases appropriate medical treatment and therapy were reactivated to restore patients to their previous profile level.

Follow-up visits often uncovered psychosocial problems within the family as a result of the chronic poststroke condition. Although the continuing medical care was adequate, there were no real guidelines for the long-term management of hemiplegia. A pilot study was under way at the time of this study to address some of these issues on a broader basis.

The authors conclude that malocclusion as a result of facial palsies can result in malnutrition, and that failure to recognize a postapoplectiform seizure often leads to unnecessary hospitalization and leaves the condition uncontrolled. Other conclusions are that the recovery of function in the upper and lower extremities varies inversely with the degree of spasticity, and that the prognosis for ambulation is equally poor in patients with right and left hemisensory loss.

> *Reviewers' Comments:* The only value of this study to occupational therapy is the conclusions drawn that offer baseline data on the recovery patterns of stroke patients, and the questions raised on splints and slings.

**52**  Mossman PL, Kerr M, Stever R

CODES:
P-2; T-4; S-1, 12,
19, 34, 40; M-2,
7, 13

## HOSPITAL UTILIZATION IN THE REHABILITATION OF COMPLETED STROKE
*Minnesota Medicine,* Jul 1977, pp 498-502

A retrospective study of the hospital records of 214 stroke patients who received comprehensive rehabilitation at the Sister Kenny Institute in the period 1970-1973 was conducted to determine the number of hospital days expended to attain a specific discharge status. The study population was carefully screened to eliminate the most and least serious cases.

Of this selected population 37 percent achieved independent status, 38.3 percent achieved semi-independent status, and 24.7 percent remained dependent or had no rehabilitation potential. The average length of hospitalization for the combined acute and rehabilitative phases of treatment was 10.5 weeks. The median total hospitalization time for the patients discharged as independent was sixty-one days for combined acute and rehabilitative care. The length of hospital stay for the more dependent patients, and therefore the more seriously impaired initially, was greater. Age was an important variable. Those who became independent were an average of 6.2 years younger than those who did not, and those who could return home were an average of 6.3 years younger than those going to nursing homes.

The rehabilitation potential of the younger stroke patient is further substantiated by this study. The authors support the philosophy of rehabilitation as a part of the treatment program for hemiplegia, not as an afterthought. Allowing the stroke patient to function at his or her maximum potential makes good medical and fiscal sense, and the length of intensive treatment needed for this must be recognized and officially sanctioned.

> *Reviewers' Comments:*
> Because this study was based on a highly selective group of patients at one facility, generalizations are invalid. However, the authors do make a reasonable argument for lengthening the period of intensive rehabilitation to ensure maximum independence and optimum results with stroke patients. They also raise pertinent questions regarding the cost effectiveness of different treatment settings, provided that the quality of care is equal across settings.

# 53 Muller EA

CODES:
P-4; T-7; S-1;
M-1, 7, 8, 13, 14

## INFLUENCE OF TRAINING AND OF INACTIVITY ON MUSCLE STRENGTH

*Archives of Physical Medicine and Rehabilitation* 51:449-462, 1970

This review evaluates the research of numerous physiologists on muscle strength, activity level, and muscle training. Muscle strength, defined as the maximum force that can be exerted against an immovable resistance by a single contraction, can be developed through various training methods designed to improve muscle function, such as isometric, concentric, isotonic, and auxotonic. The maximum strength of a muscle attainable by continued training is called limiting strength. Limiting strength increases as a function of growth in childhood and stabilizes in adulthood. The state of training of a muscle can be expressed as a percentage of its limiting strength. With maximum exercise, strength can be increased at the rate of 12 percent per week, increasing nearly linearly up to 75 percent. Above 75 percent, the rate of increase diminishes progressively to become zero at peak strength. This curve is similar for all persons, ages, sexes, and muscles. In the absence of any contraction, strength decreases by about 5 percent per day. Once attained, limiting strength can be maintained indefinitely by only one maximum contraction every two weeks in addition to usual daily activities. To assess the relative rate of strength and the maximum strength achievable from muscle training, the state of training must first be measured.

Research indicates that isometric exercise produces the greatest muscle tension with the least amount of energy expended. The influence of maximum contractions, motivation, immobility, and endurance on muscle strength is also noted. Muscles long paralyzed and atrophied retain their potential for self-regeneration through training.

*Reviewers' Comments:* This evaluation has multiple implications for occupational therapy. First, the efficiency of isometric training could be valuable for elderly or paretic patients, or for patients with cardiovascular or pulmonary problems. Second, the article demonstrates that a muscle with only one insertion intact, as in the case of an amputee, can be "trained" to increase muscle strength. Third, only limited duration of training is necessary to gain in strength if maximum resistance is used. Additional strength cannot be obtained until twenty-four hours have passed.

(continued on next page)

> Fourth, everyday activities are not sufficient to maintain the strength essential for robust health. However, very little time and energy are required to develop and maintain satisfactory strength to avoid deconditioned states.

# 54

Murray SK, Garraway WM,
Akhtar AJ, Prescott RJ

CODES:
P-2; T-3; S-1, 7,
19, 34, 40; M-1,
7, 10, 13

## COMMUNICATION BETWEEN HOME AND HOSPITAL IN THE MANAGEMENT OF ACUTE STROKE IN THE ELDERLY: RESULTS FROM A CONTROLLED TRIAL

*Health Bulletin* 40:214-219, 1982

A randomized, controlled trial in the United Kingdom compared the management of elderly patients with acute stroke in a stroke unit and in medical units. Two to three weeks after admission to the stroke unit, when the patient's condition was stabilizing, the patient and a relative were seen separately at a rehabilitation meeting. The prognosis and the plan of treatment were discussed, and the patient and the relative were given the opportunity to raise practical, social, or emotional problems.

The stroke unit increased the proportion of patients who returned to functional independence. A greater number of relatives of patients in the stroke unit reported contact with hospital staff, a higher proportion of patients had home trial visits, and more notice was given of the intention to discharge patients. The use of the rehabilitation meeting in the stroke unit was a factor in the higher level of contact. In the medical units a low level of communication with the medical consultant was reported. Communication was with the hospital's junior medical staff, concerned the patient's condition, and did not involve the family in rehabilitation. In both types of locations the satisfaction expressed by relatives about communication with hospital staff was not related to the amount of contact reported. Also in both types of locations the highest number of contacts and the greatest proportion of two-way contacts were with the ward sister, confirming her as a key person in this hospital's communication network.

*Reviewers' Comments:* The study's scientific supportability can be questioned, and somewhat superficial information is shared. However, the article offers evidence of the value of the rehabilitation stroke unit, including occupational therapy, and provides interesting observations about staff communication with patients' families.

**55** Neuhaus BE, Ascher ER, Coullon BA, Donohue MV, Einbond A, Glover JM, Goldberg SR, Takai VL

CODES: P-2; T-7; S-1, 7, 11, 21, 39; M-1, 11

# A SURVEY OF RATIONALES FOR AND AGAINST HAND SPLINTING IN HEMIPLEGIA

*American Journal of Occupational Therapy* 35:83-90, 1981

The underlying rationales of occupational therapists who make splinting decisions involving patients with hemiplegia were investigated. The survey incorporated a limited-choice, multiple-option questionnaire based on the case study of a man with a left hemiparesis at three hypothetical stages of recovery. The survey instrument was field-tested in four New York hospitals and refined before distribution to forty-two facilities in the greater New York area that treated or provided service to patients with acute and long-term neurological disorders. An 80-percent response rate was achieved.

The ninety-three occupational therapists who answered indicated whether they would recommend a splint at each stage of recovery and selected one or more reasons for their decisions. The respondents fell into three major categories: those who would never splint, those who would always splint, and those who would splint only in the presence of moderate to severe spasticity.

The respondents with more clinical experience reflected more tendency to splint. The authors conclude that there are divergent practices concerning hand splinting in hemiplegia by occupational therapists, indicating a growing need for theoretical and empirical research. The authors also summarize their review of studies covering a period of more than one hundred years and attempt to provide a historical perspective for their discussion of findings.

> *Reviewers' Comments:* The article points out the need for more research on theoretical approaches and on outcome measures when differing treatment interventions are used. It also supports the need for educational programs that encourage therapists to become aware of inconsistencies in clinical reasoning. However, this type of research may be less productive than studies that provide evidence of the effects of splinting.

**56** Pendarvis JF, Grinnell RM Jr

CODES:
P-2; T-3; S-1, 7, 19, 34, 39; M-1, 7

## THE USE OF A REHABILITATION TEAM FOR STROKE PATIENTS

*Social Work in Health Care* 6:77-85, 1980

A multidisciplinary team affiliated with a large urban hospital was evaluated with respect to its effect on stroke patients. The study sample consisted of all patients admitted to and discharged from the hospital with a diagnosis of stroke from June 1 to December 1, 1978. Patients whose hospitalization had lasted fewer than ten days were excluded. The original sample comprised eighty-five patients. Of these, thirty-seven who had been referred to the rehabilitation team during their hospitalization were considered the treatment group, and forty-eight who had not been referred to the rehabilitation team were considered the comparison group. The patients were evaluated on the basis of their scores on the Health Scale for the Aged, mailed to them three months after their discharge from the hospital. This three-question functional health scale provides self-report information on physical condition and health, sample activities, and limitations in work or activities. Of the eighty-five patients in the original population, fifty-eight responded (twenty-six from the treatment group and thirty-two from the comparison group).

Analysis of the two groups showed a significant difference in the age of the patients. The average age of the treatment group patients was 66.5 years, and the average age of the comparison group patients was 75.6 years. The average hospital stay was also significantly different--20.4 days for the treatment group, 14.2 days for the comparison group. Statistical comparison of the results of the functional health scores indicated that the patients seen by the team scored higher than those not seen by the team. The effects of age and hospital stay were removed in further statistical analysis, and a partial correlation remained statistically significant.

The authors pose some explanations for the differences and clearly identify the limitations and difficulties encountered in this type of research. They conclude that the multidisciplinary team approach as used in the hospital studied is effective in the treatment of stroke patients.

*Reviewers' Comments:* This article presents an example of a useful, simple, and straightforward design with the limitations clearly identified. It therefore may be helpful for undergraduate occupational therapy students or beginning therapists as an introduction to research and the relevance of research to occupational therapy. The conclusions support the effectiveness of the rehabilitation team. However, the design of the study imposes limitations on its reliability and validity.

# 57 Redford JB, Harris JD

CODES:
P-6, T-7; S-1, 12,
19, 34, 41; M-1,
7, 8, 13, 14

## REHABILITATION OF THE ELDERLY STROKE PATIENT

*American Family Physician* 22:153-160, 1980

A comprehensive approach to stroke management aimed at restoring patients to their fullest physical, social, vocational, and economic usefulness is discussed. The family physician plays an important role in organizing early attempts at rehabilitation and coordinating the interdisciplinary team. The characteristic deficits of stroke--the loss of motor control, a disturbed sensation, and the loss of an ability to communicate--have different implications depending on a patient's personality, life-style, attitude, and past experience. Equally important in predicting outcome are the cause, the location, and the extent of brain tissue damage; prior health status; and social status. Because rehabilitation is primarily a learning process, an evaluation of intellectual ability and emotional stability is important, as are assessments of speech, perception, motor control, and activities of daily living. A well-designed treatment program should incorporate these findings with preventive techniques, protective maneuvers, and retraining in motor and perceptual skills. Another aspect of a stroke rehabilitation program is the modification of environmental conditions to facilitate maximum independence.

*Reviewers' Comments:* This narrative, descriptive article could serve as an information resource for family members of stroke patients on the basic principles of rehabilitation. The article includes a self-care evaluation form and reinforces the role of occupational therapy in the team approach.

# 58   Robins V, Braun RM, Voss DE

CODES:
P-5; T-9; S-1, 22;
M-5, 11, 17

## SHOULD PATIENTS WITH HEMIPLEGIA WEAR A SLING?

*Physical Therapy* 49:1029-1030, 1969

Pertinent issues concerning the controversy over the use of slings by patients with hemiplegia are discussed by a physician and a physical therapist. From the physician's standpoint, a sling, like any other therapeutic device, must be used with adequate supervision. The dangers of using a sling without such supervision include dependent edema of the forearm and the hand, and adducted, internally rotated, and symptomatic shoulders. According to the physical therapist, a group of her colleagues queried during an exercise project in 1966 agreed that the use of a sling might be indicated while subluxation at the glenohumeral joint was present. However, the group thought slings had unwanted influences. They may interfere with body image, postural support of the arm, and the development of a good gait pattern with reciprocal arm swing. They hold the arm in a flexed position, reinforcing the flexion synergy with inhibition of the triceps muscle. Slings may relieve shoulder pain, but this condition could be prevented by discontinuing three traditional practices that contribute greatly to problems of subluxation and pain: the use of pulleys, passive motion therapy without attention to the position of the scapula, and stereotyped positioning in bed without proper regard for scapulohumeral relationships.

> *Reviewers' Comments:* The article correctly implies that relevant information must be collected before the appropriateness of a sling can be determined.

**59** Rosenthal AM, Pearson L, Medenica B,
Manaster A, Smith CS

CODES:
P-2; T-5; S-1, 12,
19, 39; M-1, 7,
8, 9

## CORRELATION OF PERCEPTUAL FACTORS WITH REHABILITATION OF HEMIPLEGIC PATIENTS

*Archives of Physical Medicine and Rehabilitation* 46:461-466, 1965

The hypothesis that measures of perceptual impairment could be used to predict which hemiplegic patients would benefit most from rehabilitation was examined. All patients admitted to a comprehensive rehabilitation center over a two-year period who had left hemiplegia and also had normal intelligence were evaluated. The study population comprised twenty-eight men and twenty-one women, aged twenty-five to eighty-three years. Each patient was rated on his or her performance of common self-care activities at admission and at discharge; the score reflected the percentage of change. Visual perception was measured with the Hooper Visual Organization Test and the Benton Visual Retention Test in two parts, drawing from memory and copying a geometric form.

Despite numerous data analyses, no statistical significance was found between the amount of visual-perceptual error and the degree of rehabilitation improvement. A reexamination of the study uncovered some design flaws. Expressing rehabilitative change as a percentage penalized the high-level patient who had reached the ceiling, and rewarded the severely impaired patient who had made modest improvement.

The authors conclude that a scale must be designed that assigns equal weight to various indices of change. The Benton test involving visual-motor reproduction and retention of visual configurations measures skills that do not correlate with physical rehabilitation. However, visual organization, as manifested on the Hooper test, does approach significance. If this tendency can be established at a more significant level, the central organizing processes of visual perception can be used to predict the ultimate level of response to a rehabilitation program.

> *Reviewers' Comments:* The study reconfirms the need for appropriate methods of assessment. It also considers ethical dilemmas in treatment, although they are not discussed as such.

# 60 Shah S

CODES:
P-5; T-7; S-1, 21;
M-6, 14

## OCCUPATIONAL THERAPY FOR MOTOR RE-EDUCATION OF HEMIPLEGICS

In *Proceedings of the 2nd International Congress on Muscle Diseases*, BA Kakulas, Editor. Amsterdam, The Netherlands: Excerpta Medica, 1971, part 2, pp 682-685

This article, classified as an opinion statement, presents a subjective discussion of the recovery process in hemiplegia and the role of occupational therapy in motor reeducation. The recovery process in hemiplegia generally has an orderly pattern, which should be followed in treatment planning. Early efforts should concentrate on the specific restitution of movement patterns, pregait training, bicycle pedaling using a bicycle fret saw, or propelling a wheelchair. Restitution of the arm is divided into two components, gross arm control and hand control, and should begin with flexion and extension patterns. Unilateral tasks are suggested that incorporate verbal commands, proprioceptive stimuli, and tonic reflexes for elicitation of patterns. Assistance by the unaffected arm is to be avoided. However, should there be visual field deficits, apraxia, or sensory deficits, treatment should be modified. Additional techniques to use in cases of secondary shoulder problems and/or a flaccid upper extremity are discussed briefly. Procedures used to facilitate hand control are outlined, as are various wrist and finger exercises. The author concludes that, when begun early, occupational therapy will reduce or reverse secondary changes that could interfere with the recovery of voluntary motion.

> *Reviewers' Comments:*
> Procedures are described clearly.
> However, there is no evidence to
> show that they are effective, nor is
> there a representation of other
> viewpoints. The presentation is
> also somewhat controversial in
> terms of current practice.

**61** Shah SK, Corones J

CODES:
P-2; T-5; S-1, 6,
12, 15, 21, 34,
40; M-1, 7, 8

# VOLITION FOLLOWING HEMIPLEGIA

*Archives of Physical Medicine and Rehabilitation* 61:523-528,
1980

A clinical study was undertaken to examine the paralyzed upper
extremity of 100 adult patients with hemiplegia due to a
cerebrovascular accident (CVA). Over a period of three years 105
patients were examined during the eleventh and twelfth weeks
after the onset of stroke. Five were eliminated from the study
because they did not meet established criteria. The patients who
were selected had hemiplegia due to CVAs, were capable of
understanding English, were oriented as to time and place, and
did not demonstrate a thalamic pain phenomenon in the upper
extremity that would prevent examination. Fifty patients were
males and 50 were females. Ages ranged from 49 to 88 years,
with a median age of 68.7 years. Forty-nine patients had left
CVAs, and 51 had right CVAs. The examination consisted of a
detailed assessment of the paralyzed upper extremity, including
voluntary motion, the presence of synergistic patterns, isolated
muscle function, and functional performance. Frequency
distributions, correlation coefficients, and Kendall rank-order
correlation coefficients were computed.

Forearm supination and the spontaneity of arm usage appeared
to be the best predictors of other synergistic components. The
isolated muscle function revealed during the execution of
functional tasks showed that grasping an object was the least-
affected task and dropping a coin in a slot was the most difficult.

An inability to perform voluntary motion was primarily related to the limitation of active and passive motion of the shoulders, the elbow, the wrist, and the hand. The authors speculate that a well-planned and effective occupational therapy program that translates movement learned in physical therapy would help prevent secondary changes and enhance function.

> *Reviewers' Comments:* The authors suggest that occupational therapists have a role, but the suggestion is speculative and not based on the data presented.

**62** Sheikh K, Meade TW, Brennan PJ, Goldenberg E, Smith DS

CODES: P-2; T-5; S-1, 16, 19, 34, 40; M-7, 8, 9

## INTENSIVE REHABILITATION AFTER STROKE: SERVICE IMPLICATIONS

*Community Medicine* 3:210-216, 1981

The medical records of 1,094 patients with confirmed stroke admitted to Northwick Park Hospital, London, between October 1972 and September 1978 were examined to determine how many would meet the eligibility requirements for participation in a rigorous rehabilitation program. Of the 502 male subjects, 80 met the qualifications; of the 592 female subjects, only 41 did so. Major reasons for exclusion were early death (33 percent), early functional recovery (20 percent), and old age and frailty (20 percent). Many patients were ineligible for more than one reason. Therefore, of the initial 1,094 patients considered, only 11 percent could have participated in the intensive outpatient rehabilitation program.

The authors conclude that although an earlier study (see abstract no. 63) demonstrated intensive outpatient rehabilitation after stroke to be effective in restoring independence, the demand for this kind of management has been exaggerated. The service implications of this finding should be considered in proposals relating to the use of personnel and facilities.

*Reviewers' Comments:* The authors established criteria for exclusion from the study, but made an unjustifiable assumption: that eligibility for the trial was, for all practical intents and purposes, the same as for ordinary outpatient rehabilitation. The data do not support this assumption.

**63** Smith DS, Goldenberg E, Ashburn A, Kinsella G, Sheikh K, Brennan PJ, Meade TW, Zutshi DW, Perry JD, Reeback JS

CODES:
P-2; T-3; S-1, 10, 16, 21, 22, 24, 34, 40; M-1, 7, 8, 13, 14

## REMEDIAL THERAPY AFTER STROKE: A RANDOMIZED CONTROLLED TRIAL

*British Medical Journal* 282:517-520, 1981

The effectiveness of three intensities of outpatient rehabilitation in the treatment of patients with confirmed stroke was compared. A total of 1,094 patients admitted to Northwick Park (a London district general hospital) from October 1972 to September 1978 were considered for study. Patients who had died or made a full recovery were excluded from further study. The remaining patients were screened to determine if they could manage the most intensive of the treatment regimens. A total of 121 patients (11 percent of the original population) plus 12 additional recruited patients were randomly assigned to one of three groups. Group I (46 patients, mean age sixty-three years, 67 percent males) received treatment described as "intensive," four full days a week in the rehabilitation department. Group II (43 patients, mean age sixty-six years, 73 percent males) received "conventional" treatment, three half-days per week. Group III (44 patients, mean age sixty-five years, 59 percent males) received no routine rehabilitation but were regularly seen at home by home health care visitors and were referred to the hospital as needed. These patients were also encouraged to continue with exercises taught to them while they were in the hospital. All the patients were assessed shortly after discharge on activities of daily living and were reassessed at three-, six-, and twelve-month intervals.

The data collected after three and twelve months indicated that outpatient rehabilitation after stroke was effective. Improvement was greatest for those receiving intensive treatment (Group I), intermediate for those receiving conventional treatment (Group II), and least for those receiving no routine treatment (Group III). "Spontaneous" improvement was shown in Group III. The findings further suggested that the decreasing intensity of treatment was associated with a significant increase in the proportion of patients who deterioriated and in the extent to which they deterioriated. The beneficial effects of treatment were almost entirely achieved in the first three months and were largely maintained, though not increased, during the rest of the first year.

This was chiefly a trial of different intensities of the same treatment, not a trial of qualitatively different treatments. Therefore, the authors draw no conclusions as to which parts of the overall regimen were responsible for the observed improvement apparently associated with active treatment.

NOTE: An Efficacy Data Brief on this article is available from the American Occupational Therapy Association, Quality Assurance Division.

> *Reviewers' Comments:* This study supports the benefits of outpatient rehabilitation. An important finding is that the beneficial effects of treatment are concentrated in the first three months.

**64** Smith ME, Garraway WM, Smith DL, Akhtar AJ

CODES:
P-2; T-3; S-1, 7, 21, 22, 34, 40; M-2, 7, 8, 9, 13, 14

# THERAPY IMPACT ON FUNCTIONAL OUTCOME IN A CONTROLLED TRIAL OF STROKE REHABILITATION

*Archives of Physical Medicine and Rehabilitation* 63:21-24, 1982

In this randomized controlled trial of management of acute stroke in the elderly, the use of occupational therapy and physical therapy in relation to activities of daily living (ADL) and neurological impairment was analyzed. A total of 155 patients in a rehabilitation unit and 152 patients in a medical unit were studied. The mean age of survivors was 72.5 years. Forty-seven percent of the population were males, and 53 percent were females. Data on therapy were collected retrospectively from occupational therapy and physical therapy records. The outcome of rehabilitation was assessed by neurological and ADL testing at discharge from the hospital or at sixteen weeks after admission.

Sixty-two percent of the patients in the stroke unit were assessed as independent in self-care, compared with 45 percent of the patients in the medical unit who had similar levels of neurological impairment. The patients in the stroke unit received less therapy over a shorter period; however, a higher proportion had occupational therapy much sooner after admission. The authors conclude that the early introduction of rehabilitation by therapists may be more important than the amount or the duration of treatment, particularly in occupational therapy.

NOTE: An Efficacy Data Brief on this article is available from the American Occupational Therapy Association, Quality Assurance Division.

*Reviewers' Comments:* This excellent, well-written article contributes evidence to support both the role of occupational therapists in the treatment of stroke and the use of a team approach. It also provides a discussion of the methodological issues involved in evaluating therapy services.

**65** Smith ME, Walton MS, Garraway WM

CODES: P-2; T-3; S-1, 10, 19, 34, 40; M-1, 7, 11, 13, 17, 18

# THE USE OF AIDS AND ADAPTATIONS IN A STUDY OF STROKE REHABILITATION
*Health Bulletin* 39:98-106, 1981

The provision of aids and adaptations to elderly stroke patients and the relationship of the use of aids to the achievement of independence in self-care were studied. Data were gathered from discharge evaluations, patients' relatives, and community-based occupational therapists, on 311 patients who had received rehabilitation services through a stroke unit or medical units. A total of 101 stroke unit patients and 91 medical unit patients had survived for at least one year after discharge and were available for an activities-of-daily-living evaluation. The overall distribution of patients by age and sex was similar in the stroke and medical unit groups.

The patients in the stroke unit group had been given more aids while in the hospital, had achieved greater independence at the time of discharge, and continued to use more aids one year after discharge than the medical unit patients. The use of aids did not appear to affect the level of independence achieved. At one year after discharge, patients from the medical units had reached the same level of independence as patients from the stroke unit had. The number of aids still in use was proportional to the number given during hospitalization. The highest proportion of aids given was, in the hospital, mobility aids, and after discharge, bathing aids. Feeding aids showed the greatest decrease in use after discharge. The authors conclude that, in general, patients' needs were appropriately assessed and aids were delivered promptly.

*Reviewers' Comments:* Major design flaws threaten the study's internal and external validity. However, the study provides basic information on the types of aids provided for and used by cerebrovascular accident patients and highlights the need for appropriate monitoring and follow-up. The study also provides support for the role of community-based occupational therapists.

# 66 Snook JH

CODES:
P-5; T-7; S-1, 8, 21,
38; M-1, 11, 17

## SPASTICITY REDUCTION SPLINT

*American Journal of Occupational Therapy* 33:648-651, 1979

This article, an information resource, describes the construction and the application of the Spasticity Reduction Splint, a variation of a dorsal resting hand splint that is designed to reduce spasticity and normalize tone. The theoretical basis for the splint's design was the Bobath approach of normalizing tone by using reflex-inhibiting movement patterns to prevent or inhibit abnormal postural patterns of extensor and flexor spasticity. The reflex-inhibiting movement patterns considered in the design included wrist extension, thumb extension, and finger abduction with extension of the interphalangeal joints. The Dorsal Platform Splint with Palmar Finger Pan was modified by increasing the pan width and applying finger separators to achieve abduction.

The Spasticity Reduction Splint was applied to eighteen hemiplegic or brain-damaged patients with tone ranging from mild to severe. Immediate and marked reduction of tone in the hand as well as in the entire upper extremity was observed in all cases. Patients reported the splint position to be comfortable and were pleased with its effect in reducing spasticity and the associated discomfort. Wearing time of the splint played an important role in the effectiveness of tone reduction. Splints used in two case studies are discussed.

*Reviewers' Comments:* This article suggests a possible approach to the treatment of spasticity. The study itself makes a contribution to occupational therapy for the following reasons: Improvement was shown in all cases; patients were satisfied; the splint could be independently applied; the splint's effects carried over to nonsplint time; wearing time was gradually reduced; and therapists were

(continued on next page)

enthusiastic about the device. However, contraindications and unintended side effects are not reported.

**67** Stern PH, McDowell F, Miller JM, Robinson M

CODES:
P-2; T-3; S-1, 12, 19, 33, 39; M-1, 7, 8, 14

# EFFECTS OF FACILITATION EXERCISE TECHNIQUES IN STROKE REHABILITATION

*Archives of Physical Medicine and Rehabilitation* 51:526-531, 1970

Improvements in a group of stroke patients who received a specific exercise program using neuromuscular reeducation techniques were compared with improvements in a control group whose treatment program did not include the exercises under study. Fifty stroke patients admitted to Burke Rehabilitation Center in 1968-1969 were randomly divided into two groups. Twelve patients were added to the study to equalize differences in patient characteristics in the original sample. Both groups had nineteen males and twelve females, seventeen left hemiplegics and fourteen right hemiplegics. The groups had mean ages close to sixty-four years and were alike in major clinical characteristics. They were evaluated using objective, quantitative tests of motility and strength developed at the Center. A numerical self-care scoring system (the Kenny Rehabilitation Institute Self-Care Evaluation) was used to assess functional improvement). The test battery was applied at weekly intervals, but only the values obtained at admission and discharge were used in the statistical comparison of the two groups.

Improvements on the three measures were seen in both groups. The differences between the groups were not significant. The authors suggest that a therapeutic program using facilitation exercises as outlined in this study does not significantly improve the motility and strength deficits observed in this patient population.

*Reviewers' Comments:* The validity of the study is at issue. However, the article presents some implications for occupational therapy. It raises the question as to which form of treatment is the most efficacious and suggests that the most efficacious treatment is not always the most "innovative." Until unquestionable evidence is presented for a treatment of choice, alternative management techniques should be viewed with caution.

## 68

Stern PH, McDowell F, Miller JM, Robinson M

CODES:
P-2; T-3; S-1, 12, 19, 33, 39; M-1, 7, 8, 13, 14

## FACTORS INFLUENCING STROKE REHABILITATION

*Stroke* 2:213-218, 1971

Clinical evaluations of sixty-two stroke patients admitted to the Burke Rehabilitation Center in 1968 and 1969 were conducted and analyzed. The patients were the subjects of an earlier statistical analysis by the same authors of the effects of differing therapeutic exercise regimens for stroke patients (see abstract no. 67). Because improvements made by each group were not significantly different, the data were pooled and analyzed to discern patterns of recovery and to weigh the influence of various factors on recovery. Assessments included motility studies, leg strength measurements, sensory testing, and functional status evaluations. Factors analyzed included the effect of facilitation exercises, the severity of paresis, the interval between the onset of stroke and rehabilitation, and the effect of hemisensory loss on self-care status.

Improvement in motility and leg strength was minimal and was not influenced by facilitation exercise techniques. The patients with short intervals between onset and admission improved significantly more; little neurological change was observed after two months. Despite relatively static neurological deficits, all patients showed evidence of functional improvement on a self-care rating scale. Those with hemisensory losses in addition to motor deficits, however, improved the least. Hemiparetic patients achieved a higher level of self-care function in about half the hospital stay, compared with hemiplegic patients. The observations made in this study support early rational and functionally oriented stroke rehabilitation programs.

> *Reviewers' Comments:*
> Although the subject matter of this article relates to rehabilitation and occupational therapy, the article itself lacks sufficient documentation of the treatment methods used and the intervention provided to assess the validity and the reliability of the results.

**69** Stonnington HH

CODES:
P-6; T-7; S-1,19;
M-1,5,7,8,9,10

## REHABILITATION IN CEREBROVASCULAR DISEASES

*Primary Care* 7:87-106, 1980

Information is provided on the comprehensive rehabilitation effort required if stroke patients are to achieve maximum functional potential. The material is organized into four parts: a detailed evaluation of the patient and his or her environment, an evaluation of the patient's potential for rehabilitation and the setting of goals, management of rehabilitation as demonstrated in three case studies, and a diagram of the many factors involved in the rehabilitation equation for a stroke patient. A distinction is made between teaching the patient to compensate for lost functions and restoring lost functions, or rehabilitation. The basis for a rehabilitative approach in this article is the plasticity of the central nervous system, which enables the brain to restore or reroute destroyed pathways, as long as functional use is stimulated and demanded. Because rehabilitation is more timely and costly and takes the expertise of more professionals than a compensatory approach, it is important to assess the realistic potential of a patient before structuring the therapeutic program. Guidelines are offered for making a prognosis based on evaluations of a patient's excretory function, mental status, sensory picture, level of communication, motor skills, and pain. Rehabilitation goals focus on mobility, activities of daily living, vocational planning, homemaking, recreation, and the ability to love and be loved. The ultimate aim is to allow the patient to live with the maximum amount of dignity and independence and with the best quality of life that is available under the circumstances.

> *Reviewers' Comments:* This article provides a general and basic overview of the components of a comprehensive stroke evaluation, the factors to consider in treatment planning, the value of teamwork, and the appropriate involvement of occupational therapists in the rehabilitation of stroke patients. The content is particularly well suited to students, as part of their professional education curriculum.

**70**  Tan ES, Don RG

CODES:
P-2; T-6; S-1, 6,
19, 34, 40; M-2,
7, 8, 11

# REHABILITATION OF CEREBROVASCULAR DISEASE WITH NEUROLOGICAL DEFICITS--RESULTS OF 500 CASES TREATED BETWEEN 1973 & 1978

*Singapore Medical Journal* 22:210-213, 1981

Five hundred consecutive cases of cerebrovascular disease with neurological deficits treated at Tan Tock Seng Hospital in Singapore between 1973 and 1978 were reviewed. Of the sample 60.2 percent were males and 43.6 percent were older than sixty years of age. There was an almost equal distribution of left and right hemiplegics. Eight of the subjects had had bilateral strokes. Ninety-four percent stayed in the hospital less than three months. Seventy-nine percent achieved total independence in self-care activities, and about seventeen percent gained partial independence. More than 90 percent were able to ambulate with or without aids at the time of discharge from the hospital. Of the 229 who were employed at the time of stroke, 108 were able to return to gainful employment. Of the 66 housewives, 44 were able to resume the performance of household chores after discharge. The authors conclude that early rehabilitation provides the patient with a better chance for recovery.

> *Reviewers' Comments:* The article provides a detailed analysis of the characteristics of the study population and describes the functional status of the group after rehabilitation. However, the study is not clearly defined, and threats to its internal and external validity are evident.

# 71 Trombly CA

CODES:
P-2; T-3; S-1, 21,
34, 38; M-1, 8, 14

## EFFECTS OF SELECTED ACTIVITIES ON FINGER EXTENSION OF ADULT HEMIPLEGIC PATIENTS

*American Journal of Occupational Therapy* 18:233-239, 1964

This study was undertaken to gather objective data on the effects of various treatment procedures on finger extension. An examination of neurophysiological theory noted four responses basic to manual dexterity: stretch, resistance, grasp, and isotonic contraction. A clinical trial was designed. Eight male stroke patients, four with right hemiparesis and four with left, participated in the study. Six subjects were treated for two consecutive five-day periods, and two subjects were treated for one five-day period. During the first period each subject performed one of four activities to which he had been randomly assigned. During the second five-day period each performed a different activity. The activities were as follows: flicking lightweight balls into a target, a light phasic activity of the finger extensors; static grasping of two differently shaped handles; puzzle making, a grasp-release activity; and using an exercise glove that gave direct resistance to the finger extensors, a heavy phasic activity. To evaluate the neuromuscular integration of finger extension, the subjects' range of motion, balance of muscle tone, gross manual dexterity, and strength of finger extension of the involved and uninvolved hands were measured before and after daily treatment.

All of the activities improved strength. Positive effects on the neuromuscular integration of finger extension resulted from heavy and light phasic activities and from static grasp. The author believes that a more thorough investigation, along with refinement in the measurement techniques, is warranted. Because of the small study population, the brevity of the observation period, and the heterogeneity of the patient group, the findings are considered merely indicative of trends.

> ***Reviewers' Comments:*** The research is not current, but, in general, this is a potentially useful pilot study suggesting possible directions for further research of a more valid and reliable nature and offering hypotheses that need to be tested in additional studies.

**72**  Truscott BL, Kretschmann CM, Toole JF, Pajak TF

CODES:
P-2; T-3; S-1, 6,19, 34, 40; M-2,7, 8, 14

# EARLY REHABILITATIVE CARE IN COMMUNITY HOSPITALS: EFFECT ON QUALITY OF SURVIVORSHIP FOLLOWING A STROKE

*Stroke* 5:623-629, 1974

The effects of the early institution of rehabilitative care on the quality of survivorship were investigated in 483 patients with their first cerebral infarction. The patients were treated under the North Carolina Comprehensive Stroke Program. Instituted in twenty-five community hospitals that had little or no specialized rehabilitative personnel and equipment (they were present in only three of the twenty-five hospitals), the program provided uniform instruction in diagnosis, evaluation, and treatment of stroke patients. Uniform guidelines were applied in evaluation of weakness, functional capacity, and levels of consciousness. Data from medical histories and treatment were recorded and entered into a master computer file. Consequently a homogeneous well-defined data base was available to the authors to study the effects of early institution of care on mortality and the return of motor function during the first three months following stroke.

The 483 patients were grouped according to age, state of consciousness at the onset of stroke, and presence of associated diseases. Cohorts were divided into those receiving no rehabilitation and those receiving a program of passive range of motion and positioning within forty-eight hours of onset. The common denominator was the early institution of rehabilitation according to uniform guidelines.

The factor most indicative of a favorable outcome was the state of consciousness at admission. Impaired consciousness resulted in a mortality rate four times greater than that of individuals who remained alert and aware. Improvement in motor strength was also much lower for patients with impaired consciousness. The presence of hypertension did not affect mortality appreciably, but early rehabilitation positively reduced the in-hospital death rate of hypertensive patients as well as those with other coexisting diseases.

*Reviewers' Comments:* The validity of this study is debatable. The article's main contribution is its support of early rehabilitation. However, "early rehabilitation" as used in the article does not specifically include occupational therapy. The majority of the hospitals did not have specialized rehabilitation personnel, even though the phrase "allied health personnel" is used in the description of the methodology.

# 73  Wade DT, Skilbeck CE, Hewer RL

CODES:
P-2; T-5; S-1, 6,
19, 34, 40; M-1,
7, 8

## PREDICTING BARTHEL ADL SCORE AT 6 MONTHS AFTER AN ACUTE STROKE

*Archives of Physical Medicine and Rehabilitation* 64:24-27, 1983

The problem of predicting the outcome of a stroke was addressed. Prediction was based on a patient's activities-of-daily-living (ADL) score at a fixed interval after stroke using data available shortly after the onset of stroke. Of a total study base of 162 referred patients, 83 comprised the selected study population. Nearly equal numbers of males and females were included; their mean age was 66.5 years. Multiple regression was used to identify five variables that had been measured at initial assessment and that correlated with the Barthel score six months after stroke. These variables were age, hemianopia or visual inattention, urinary incontinence, motor deficit in the affected arm, and sitting balance. The combined correlation of the five variables with the Barthel score at six months was 0.62.

The equation derived from the five variables successfully predicted the Barthel ADL score in 55 percent of the surviving patients. A second equation that was developed provided less accurate predictions. The authors conclude that the initial equation incorporating the five variables provides a better predictor of six-month status than can be achieved through other methods, including adding the average improvement to a patient's initial Barthel score. They recommend that future research focus on predicting a patient's status at a set time rather than attempting to predict changes over time.

> *Reviewers' Comments:* The study needs to be cross-validated before results can be generalized. Methodological flaws include the type of regression analysis chosen and the use of the same patient group to develop and test a prediction equation. The study
> (continued on next page)

does suggest an area of research appropriate for occupational therapists, namely, the predictability of functional gain.

**74** Warren M

CODES:
P-2; T-5; S-1, 12,
21, 34, 40; M-1,
7, 8

## RELATIONSHIP OF CONSTRUCTIONAL APRAXIA AND BODY SCHEME DISORDERS TO DRESSING PERFORMANCE IN ADULT CVA

*American Journal of Occupational Therapy* 35:431-437, 1981

The relationship of constructional apraxia and body scheme disorders to the failure of cerebrovascular accident (CVA) patients to achieve independence in upper extremity dressing was investigated. The study sample consisted of 101 inpatients at the Rehabilitation Institute of Kansas City between July 1978 and December 1979. The criteria for selecting subjects included a minimum age of thirteen years, a diagnosis of CVA with evidence of unilateral lesions, an ability to participate in evaluations, and an ability to perform writing tasks on command. There were 54 left CVAs (32 males and 22 females), with a mean age of 64.11 years, and 47 right CVAs (23 males and 24 females), with a mean age of 74.61 years. Subjects were given tests that measured body scheme dysfunction and constructional apraxia on admission to the inpatient rehabilitation unit. They were then rated on upper-extremity dressing performance at discharge.

Scores on the apraxia and body scheme tests were statistically correlated with ratings on dressing performance. The results indicated that both constructional apraxia and body scheme dysfunction were related to failure to achieve upper extremity dressing. Body scheme performance was a better predictor of dressing ability than constructional apraxia was. Visual field deficits, medical complications, and aphasia exerted a significant influence on patients' performance. The right CVA group contained a significantly greater proportion of dressing failures and visual field deficits. Aphasia appeared to play a significant role in the performance of the left CVA group. A subject's disability and number of complications during recovery also significantly influenced ultimate achievement in dressing. The author proposes that simple clinical tests may be used to predict the potential of a patient to benefit from dressing training.

> *Reviewers' Comments:* The scientific supportability of the research is debatable. The data offer evidence that constructional apraxia and body scheme have a relationship to dressing performance, but not one of cause and effect.

**75** Weisbroth S, Esibill N, Zuger RR

CODES:
P-2; T-4; S-1, 12, 20, 33, 39; M-2, 7, 8, 9

## FACTORS IN THE VOCATIONAL SUCCESS OF HEMIPLEGIC PATIENTS

*Archives of Physical Medicine and Rehabilitation* 52:441-446, 486; 1971

Vocational, demographic, physical-function, and cognitive variables were examined in a group of hemiplegic patients under age sixty-five. The study was undertaken to determine why some hemiplegic patients seen for vocational counseling returned to work whereas others did not, despite comparable medical and vocational rehabilitation efforts. The patients selected for the study were sixty-two who had attended more than one vocational counseling session at the Institute of Rehabilitation Medicine between July 1, 1965, and June 30, 1969. Included were forty-three males and nineteen females, thirty-four right hemiplegics and twenty-eight left hemiplegics.

More than one-third of the patients returned to work, more women than men. Variables that significantly differentiated left hemiplegic returnees from nonreturnees included ambulation, use of the affected upper extremity, and nonverbal abstract reasoning. Variables that significantly differentiated right hemiplegic returnees from nonreturnees revolved around a marked verbal cognitive and communicative deficit. Analysis of speech problems in right hemiplegics yielded a significant difference between returnees and nonreturnees in scores on the Functional Communication Profile. The length of time between the onset of disability and the return to a vocation averaged 15.7 months for right hemiplegics, 19.2 for left hemiplegics. The authors recommend more emphasis on learning principles, on-the-job training, cognitive retraining, modifications of situations, and careful vocational planning in total rehabilitation efforts.

> *Reviewers' Comments:*
> Samples sizes are small, and the reader is cautioned against generalizations and stereotyping of patients. However, the article provides perspectives on vocational rehabilitation that warrant consideration in team management.

# 76

Wolcott LE, Wheeler PC, Ballard P, Crumb CK, Miles G, Mueller A

CODES: P-2; T-7; S-1, 8, 10, 19, 33, 34, 39; M-1, 7, 10, 13

## HOME-CARE VS. INSTITUTIONAL REHABILITATION OF STROKE: A COMPARATIVE STUDY

*Missouri Medicine* 63:722-724, 1966

The effectiveness of home care and institutional rehabilitation of stroke patients was compared, using restoration of independent functional abilities as the chief criterion. The population consisted of thirty-nine patients who received rehabilitative care in an institution and seventeen patients who received rehabilitative care at home from a trained nurse supervised by a family physician. A survey form was devised to compile patient information on demographic and medical factors, proficiency in activities of daily living (ADL), psychosocial status, and opinions regarding the rehabilitation services.

Results indicated that the programs achieved the same degree of functional restoration. The average motivation for rehabilitation was identical for the two groups, and motivation correlated directly with progress in functional ability. Patients who had a high opinion of the rehabilitation program in which they participated were also highly motivated for rehabilitation. In both programs there appeared to have been an advantage in starting rehabilitation as soon as possible after the acute phase of stroke had subsided. However, two factors favored the home care program. First, the home care group achieved the same degree of proficiency in performing ADL despite being an average of ten years older. Second, in patients with marginal motivation the home care program seemed to have had a decided advantage, perhaps because the home care nurse was available to advise and counsel the family. Also, the regression that could occur following institutional discharge was not a factor. The authors conclude that in light of overtaxed facilities, personnel shortages, and rising costs, home care rehabilitation services deserve attention.

*Reviewers' Comments:*
Although the study is nearly twenty years old and statistically weak, the findings show that home care for stroke patients is as effective as institutional care in the restoration of ADL. The rehabilitation care identified in the article would be provided today by occupational therapy personnel rather than by nurses.

**77** Wolf SL, Baker MP, Kelly JL

CODES:
P-2; T-2; S-1, 16, 22, 33, 39;M-1, 7, 8, 14

# EMG BIOFEEDBACK IN STROKE: A 1-YEAR FOLLOW-UP ON THE EFFECT OF PATIENT CHARACTERISTICS

*Archives of Physical Medicine and Rehabilitation* 61:351-355, 1980

One-year follow-up data were compiled on the condition of twenty-eight upper and twenty-six lower extremities among thirty-four hemiplegic patients who received electromyographic (EMG) biofeedback training. This represented 65.4 percent of the original study population. Patients were reassessed at varying intervals and at one year after completion of the feedback training sessions. Changes in outcome status were computed based on one-year data. Examinations included specific muscle group assessments, passive-range-of-motion and EMG assessments, gait evaluations, hand function (for patients with previous difficulty), and interviews with family members. An outcome grading system consisting of failure, moderate, and success categories was used, based on criteria established during the original study.

Age, sex, the limbs involved, the duration of stroke or previous rehabilitation, and the number of biofeedback sessions showed no relationship to outcome variations at one-year follow-up. In general, improvements made during the original training period were retained at one year. Case summaries are provided for four patients in whom changes in outcome classification were attributed to alterations in neuromuscular status. The authors conclude that study findings are encouraging, but they recommend combining EMG with comprehensive exercise programs and evaluating the combined procedures.

*Reviewers' Comments:* The article does not provide sufficient data on the grading system to analyze the study's validity. However, the case summaries may be of interest, for they suggest the possibility of improvements in functional status after a lengthier poststroke period than is commonly believed. The article also provides useful information on EMG biofeedback as an adjunct to rehabilitation.

# 78 Yu J

CODES:
P-4; T-11; S-1;
M-5, 8, 14

## FUNCTIONAL RECOVERY WITH AND WITHOUT TRAINING FOLLOWING BRAIN DAMAGE IN EXPERIMENTAL ANIMALS: A REVIEW

*Archives of Physical Medicine and Rehabilitation* 57:38-41, 1976

This review article discusses functional recovery in experimental animals following brain damage. Observations show that some functions may recover spontaneously and that functional accomplishment can be increased by training even with an unchanged reflex status. Training consists of a combination of two basic techniques: forced use of the impaired body part, and instrumental conditional reflexes. The possible mechanisms of recovery include restoration by an alternate pathway, compensation through complicated interactions among brain structures, and, with training, activation of a parallel system essential to conditioned responses. Such factors as motivation and emotion may complicate the course of recovery. The author concludes that experimental animal research findings strongly indicate that training can play an active and specific part in the recovery of function in humans after brain damage.

> ***Reviewers' Comments:***
> Relating animal research to human function for clinical applicability may not be appropriate. However, the article does offer an example of tested treatment/training strategies that support the importance of rehabilitation in functional recovery.

# THE EFFICACY OF OCCUPATIONAL THERAPY IN THE TREATMENT OF STROKE

*Susan C. Merrill, MA, OTR*

The purpose of this synthesis is to integrate the findings of thirteen articles that seem to provide the clearest understanding of the efficacy of occupational therapy practice with patients who have suffered a cerebrovascular accident. The synthesis is intended to assist occupational therapy clinicians, researchers, and administrators in developing an awareness of the nature of current research in this area.

The thirteen articles discussed here were selected from the eighty-eight originally sent to the validity panel. They were chosen according to the combined judgment of the validity panel, the project consultant, and the staff of the Quality Assurance Division of the AOTA. Some articles judged by these experts to contain information of heuristic value were included even if the internal or external validity was thought to be flawed.

A charting system was used to pull salient information from each article for comparison with other articles. The information included the size of the sample, the authors' conclusions, the setting of the study, the assessment of the validity panel, the age of the subjects, and the design of the study.

The limitations of this or any synthesis must be recognized. First, the terminology and the concepts used in the various studies selected for synthesis are not necessarily defined in the same way across the studies, conceptually or operationally. Home health care, for example, may refer in one study to an entire rehabilitation team delivering services in the home, and in another study to a nurse trained in providing techniques deemed valuable to stroke patients.

Second, an individual article's richness is sometimes lost when the article is synthesized with others. The research design, the procedures for selecting subjects, and the methods of obtaining data are not mentioned here, unless they bear significantly on the synthesis. The reader is referred to the abstracts and to the articles themselves for details on methodology.

Finally, as previously indicated, many of the articles used in this synthesis were found by the validity panel to have statistical or methodological flaws. The difficulties of conducting research in clinical settings are myriad, and issues such as matching subjects, obtaining optimal sample sizes, and controlling variables are not easy to resolve. In attempting to address important clinical questions, researchers often find adherence to a strict experimental design impossible, despite heroic efforts. In the opinion of the authors of this publication, the articles synthesized here contain useful ideas and conclusions despite potential or actual methodological flaws. An additional justification for inclusion of these articles lies in the purpose of this synthesis. To illustrate the current status of research on the efficacy of occupational therapy with stroke patients, the best of the existing articles must be discussed, whether or not they meet preestablished criteria of excellence. Fruitful areas in which deficiencies might be remedied and additional research might be conducted are discussed at the end of this synthesis.

## SPECIFIC TREATMENT TECHNIQUES

In retrieving data relevant to the efficacy of occupational therapy with stroke patients, special emphasis was placed on locating articles discussing specific treatment techniques used by occupational therapists. Such specific techniques and approaches include splinting, neuromuscular facilitation, functional activity training, and therapeutic exercise. No efficacy data were found regarding specific techniques used by a therapist to assist patients in the improvement--or the attainment--of skills for relevant occupations. However, several articles documenting studies that attempted to predict functional outcomes by assessing and treating perceptual and motor skills are of interest. These articles illustrate an approach to the treatment of stroke patients that can be used in occupational therapy.

An article by Bell, Jurek, and Wilson (1) discusses the development of hand skills in hemiplegic patients. Bell and her collaborators used a hand-skill assessment tool to predict potential for rehabilitation in the dressing element of self-maintenance. Hand skill and dressing were rated for a sample of thirty patients. The probability that those scoring above 50 on the hand skill test would succeed in learning to dress was .98, indicating that the scale could be used to predict with an extremely high degree of accuracy, subjects who would learn to dress.

As a result of this finding, Bell and her colleagues altered the treatment approach for stroke patients receiving occupational therapy in their facility. Patients scoring below 50 on the hand skill assessment were given a brief trial of dressing training. With those for whom dressing training was unsuccessful, therapy focused instead on developing the skill of the unaffected hand. When the hand skill score of 50 was reached on reevaluation, dressing training was started again. Dressing skills were then usually learned in less than one week of treatment.

The significance of the article is twofold. First, the authors describe an instrument and a process (albeit a pilot study) that demonstrated the development of tools and methods to ensure efficacious practice. By refining the evaluation process, these authors directly influenced the quality and the cost effectiveness of therapy provided to their patients.

Second, the tool itself is a significant contribution, potentially useful in both practice and research. Assessment methods that allow a prediction of the outcome of therapy are invaluable to clinicians and researchers alike.

In a related study Warren (2) reports data on the relationship between constructional apraxia and body scheme disorders, on the one hand, and dressing performance in adult stroke patients. The findings support the contention that constructional apraxia and body scheme disorders are related to dressing apraxia in poststroke subjects. Dysfunction in both areas correlated significantly with failure to attain independence in dressing. The test of body scheme, however, was a better predictor of dressing performance than the constructional praxis test (design copy) was.

Warren's findings are significant for occupational therapy practice in that simple clinical tests were used to predict the potential of a patient to benefit from dressing training. This is similar to Bell and her collaborators' use of hand skill function to predict the success of dressing training. Warren points out that the need to identify patients who will and will not benefit from occupational therapy services becomes increasingly acute as pressures mount to curb health care costs. Furthermore, the provision of efficacious treatment necessitates the designation of patients who can and cannot benefit from therapeutic programs.

Warren also found that the right-hemisphere stroke patients in her study had more dressing failures than the members of the left hemisphere group did. More right- than left-hemisphere stroke subjects had visual field deficits. Aphasia appeared to play a significant role in the performance of subjects in the left hemisphere group. Nonaphasic subjects performed consistently better on the tests of body scheme and design copy and achieved greater independence in self-care than aphasic subjects.

Another article analyzing differences between patients having right and left hemisphere stroke is that by Diller and his colleagues (3). These authors measured activities-of-daily-living (ADL) performance, which they operationalized as transfer to and from a wheelchair. A broad range of assessment methods was used, including a battery of perceptual-motor tests (sensory tasks, motor speed, visual-motor performance, and attentional measures), a physician's rating scale, a functional communication profile, and observation of physical therapy training in transfer techniques. None of the tests seemed to evaluate body scheme or constructional praxis specifically, although they did emphasize perceptual and perceptual-motor abilities. The authors found no difference between the two groups in initial or final performance levels on the ADL task chosen.

They did, however, find different correlation factors between right- and left-hemisphere stroke patients, which led them to the conclusion that different teaching styles are appropriate for the two groups. With regard to mechanisms in right-hemisphere stroke patients, two of the findings were that correlates of ADL did not change over time and that poor performance on discrimination rather than sequencing of tasks appeared to be related to ADL performance.

For left-hemisphere stroke patients neither of the above applied. Correlates changed over time, and skills in sequential activities were more closely related to ADL performance than skills at tasks of specific discrimination.

The authors conclude that ADL performance is predictable. In their view the two best indicators of ultimate functional ability are the level of assistance initially required and the level of organicity. The authors describe organicity as certain behavioral patterns that provide the mental context for acquisition of a skill and that are commonly found in individuals with brain damage. Organicity was operationalized in the study using the various test parameters mentioned previously, as was performance on the ADL transfer.

Here, then, are three articles (1, 2, 3) that document studies attempting to look at specific perceptual and motor abilities in adult stroke patients as predictive of ability to relearn functional tasks. Data from Warren (2) and Diller et al. (3) conflicted on differences in the ability of right- and left-hemisphere stroke patients to learn ADL tasks, although both studies did note differences. The complexities of the tasks in the two studies (transferring to and from a wheelchair and dressing oneself) were vastly different. This is one of many possible reasons for the differences in the findings.

Two articles on the splinting of hemiplegic upper extremities are also noteworthy in terms of occupational therapy intervention techniques. One article (4) describes a study that compared volar and dorsal splints. Recognizing that only twenty subjects were used and that they were in no way matched for length of disability, age, or side of hemiplegia, the validation panel still felt that the article provided data of historical significance relevant to occupational therapy splinting practices. In the article the author reports that volar splints appeared to facilitate the flexor muscles and, in some cases, increase spasticity. Dorsal splints appeared to have the opposite effect, facilitating the extensor muscles. Also, constant wearing of either a dorsal or a volar splint possibly had an adverse effect, from maintaining the hand rigid for too long. The author strongly advocates regular passive exercise of the hand and wrist alternating with splint wearing. She also suggests that neuromuscular facilitation techniques be used to reinforce the facilitative effects of the dorsal splint.

The second article (5) also discusses the merits of dorsal splinting. The author, a clinician, used the case study method, documenting the reduction of spasticity in the hemiplegic upper extremity of two patients through dorsal splinting. The author states that these were preliminary findings; however, no follow-up article was found in the literature.

Neither of these studies employed methodology that allows reliable or valid conclusions to be drawn about splinting for upper extremity spasticity in hemiplegia. The articles do, however, provide historical information and indicate the possibility that splinting, in combination with range-of-motion and facilitation procedures, contributes to the regulation of abnormal tonus in the spastic, hemiplegic upper extremity. Both articles, more notably the one by Snook (5), describe techniques and treatment approaches.

# OUTCOMES OF REHABILITATION

Most of the articles reflecting the current status of occupational therapy efficacy data were found in the general rehabilitation medicine literature. For discussion purposes, these articles, all dealing with outcomes of rehabilitation, have been divided into three general groups that are not mutually exclusive. The first group consists of articles that also mention the cost effectiveness of rehabilitation. The second group comprises articles discussing outcomes of outpatient rehabilitation. The third group is made up of the remaining articles, including a series reporting different aspects of a single study conducted in Britain.

## COST EFFECTIVENESS AND OUTCOME

The cost effectiveness of stroke rehabilitation as a topic was not actively searched for this publication. Nonetheless, a few articles addressing cost effectiveness were found. The two selected for discussion here used *estimated* costs in two ways: first, to establish what institutionalization and home-care costs would have been without rehabilitation; second, and more important, to establish the costs of rehabilitation. The estimates were based on allowable Medicare reimbursement rates. As judged by the validity panel, the rationale for using estimates rather than actual costs was vague in both articles; therefore, panel members questioned this approach to cost analysis.

One of the studies, by Bryant, Candland, and Loewenstein (6), compared cost outcomes among three groups of stroke patients (fifty people altogether). One group required home care for at least one form of therapy, including occupational therapy. The second group comprised inpatients who did not receive home health care but did receive physical therapy while they were hospitalized. Other services such as occupational therapy were used in the hospital, but physical therapy was the one discipline received across all cases. The third group was composed of inpatients who received no home care and no physical or occupational therapy.

Estimated total costs for the nine-month period of the study were calculated. Costs for the home health care group were significantly less than those for the hospitalized groups. The authors found that the physical therapy group of hospitalized patients was not discharged to home because of insufficient functional status. Nursing home costs were then involved. Also, this group required an average of ten days more therapy than the home health care group required. The authors conclude that home health care greatly reduces costs and results in fewer deaths, fewer readmissions, and better-quality outcomes.

In the second article, by Lehmann et al. (7), cost-benefit factors were estimated for the rehabilitation services provided to a group of stroke patients. The data indicated that stroke rehabilitation paid for itself by allowing patients to be discharged to more desirable settings. Many patients who had been institutionalized before admission for rehabilitation were able to go home because of functional gains and to stay there at a lower cost than if long-term care in a nursing home had been needed.

Together the two studies suggest--but do not prove--that rehabilitation services can have cost-effective, positive outcomes, whether they are delivered at home or in a rehabilitation center. The articles support the contention that in the long term, rehabilitation is less expensive than institutional maintenance.

## REHABILITATION OUTCOMES FOR OUTPATIENTS

Two articles were found that contribute to an understanding of the efficacy of outpatient rehabilitation for stroke patients. Smith et al. (8) used a randomized controlled trial to look at the outcomes of outpatient rehabilitation for 133 stroke patients after hospital discharge. Three patient groups were used: those undergoing intensive rehabilitation, conventional rehabilitation, and no rehabilitation. Patients were assessed at three and twelve months, using an index of independence in activities of daily living.

The authors found that functional improvement was greatest in those receiving the intensive treatment and least in those receiving no routine treatment. The beneficial effects of treatment occurred primarily in the first three months of the outpatient programs and were largely maintained for the rest of the first year (the duration of the study).

Bryant, Candland, and Loewenstein (6), in the previously mentioned study on cost effectiveness, looked at outpatient treatment in the form of home health care. Patients were seen for therapy and training in their homes rather than being transported to a facility. As discussed earlier, the authors compared patients who received home health care, patients who received no home health care but who had received physical therapy while hospitalized, and patients who received no home health care and no physical therapy. The findings were that the group receiving home health care had the shortest original hospitalizations, the fewest readmissions for subsequent strokes, and the fewest deaths. Unfortunately, functional outcomes were not monitored. The methods of randomization and matching used in the study are not well reported in the article. That made judgments about the study's internal and external validity impossible for the validity panel.

These two articles support the potential of outpatient rehabilitation to effect positive outcomes for stroke patients. The articles also discuss the importance of the entire rehabilitation team, which in both cases included occupational therapy personnel.

## GENERAL REHABILITATION ARTICLES

Two articles discussing the effect of rehabilitation on the quality of life of stroke survivors are of interest. The first, a study by Anderson, Baldridge, and Ettinger (9), used quality assurance methods to assess outcomes for 84 patients who had received no rehabilitation. A greater percentage of these patients died, and fewer were independent in self-care, than had been predicted. The patients in this no-rehabilitation group were compared with a previously studied group of 119 who had received rehabilitation. The authors state that the group that had received rehabilitation consisted of individuals who were more severely involved than individuals in the no-rehabilitation group. This gives significance to the fact that in the rehabilitation group

69 percent were independent in self-care at follow-up, as opposed to 47 percent of the no-rehabilitation group. The authors conclude that the main effect of rehabilitation is on the quality of life following stroke, because the rehabilitation group members were more independent in self-care, more able to live at home or outside an institution, and showed a greater capacity to engage in employment, homemaking, or some type of daily activity.

Truscott et al. (10) reported similar findings. They compared two groups of patients. One received both medical care and rehabilitation services within forty-eight hours of being hospitalized following stroke, and the other received medical care but no rehabilitation services. The authors appear to have used consecutive sampling, but this is not explicitly stated. Additionally the authors do not state whether they made efforts to match subjects from each group, so the study's internal validity is unknown. The authors analyzed the outcomes of survivorship and return of motor skills at discharge and three months following discharge. They found that early rehabilitation was associated with reduced mortality and improved quality of survivorship in the stroke patients studied.

The value and the importance of early rehabilitation intervention were documented in two other articles reporting on the same study (11, 12). The authors randomly assigned three hundred patients to either a stroke unit, where full rehabilitation was received, or a medical unit. The methodology used was a randomized controlled trial, which gives confidence in the validity of the results. Patients in both types of units received occupational therapy. A higher proportion of subjects with similar neurological impairments achieved independence in the stroke unit than in medical units. The data suggested that earlier referral for therapy rather than the amount or the duration of treatment was an important factor. This applied in particular to occupational therapy. Patients in the stroke unit received less occupational therapy over a shorter period (but received it closer to their stroke) and had better functional outcomes. They had briefer hospitalizations and were more independent at discharge, as is reported in Cost Effectiveness and Outcome, above.

Some of these same authors performed a follow-up study on the patients described above, starting at hospital discharge or sixteen weeks after admission and continuing for one year (13). To the authors' surprise, the stroke unit patients did not sustain their gains in functional abilities. Furthermore, many of the medical unit patients continued to improve during the year following acute stroke, thereby becoming independent. Thus, although therapeutic intervention at an early stage after the onset of stroke created a temporary improvement in functional outcome, it did not provide a sustained advantage. The authors speculate that a primary reason for this result was poor preparation of the family before discharge. Patients who regressed from independence to dependence were more protected by family members and perhaps given more assistance than they required.

The other factor that the authors think contributed to the reported outcome was the larger number of patients from medical units who had been dependent at discharge but who had gained their independence by follow-up. This group had had a much shorter hospitalization than other medical unit patients. Consequently they had received less physical and occupational therapy. The authors postulate that for these patients, full rehabilitation potential had not been realized at hospital discharge.

The results of this follow-up study do not negate the potential functional improvement for stroke patients from full rehabilitation in a specialized unit. Rather, the results confirm those of previously mentioned studies, that stroke rehabilitation potential continues beyond the acute hospital phase. These data also suggest the need for long-term follow-up and good communication between the rehabilitation team and the family of the patient to promote long-term maintenance of functional abilities.

## IMPLICATIONS FOR RESEARCH AND QUALITY ASSURANCE STUDIES

The articles synthesized here provide a valuable overview of recent data on the efficacy of occupational therapy practice with people who have suffered a cerebrovascular accident. It is clear that very little data exist pertaining to the efficacy of specific treatment techniques and approaches used by occupational therapists. Articles that provide preliminary data on outcome prediction are very promising. However, more data are needed on splinting, dressing, feeding, and facilitation techniques, as well as on the therapeutic use of occupation. Such data are essential to the maintenance of the profession as a necessary, viable, cost-effective component of rehabilitation for stroke patients.

The articles synthesized here lend credence to the importance of stroke rehabilitation with occupational therapy as part of the team, for both inpatients and outpatients. The synthesis itself points out the need for studies that deal specifically with occupational therapy's role in rehabilitative intervention. Answers are needed to questions about the nature and the cost effectiveness of occupational therapy's contribution to the functional outcomes of rehabilitation.

In light of Medicare's Prospective Payment System and other federal measures to limit health care expenditures, there is a greater urgency than ever to maintain or improve productivity and the quality of care. Research in the form of qualitative, descriptive studies; quantitative, controlled-variable studies; and quality assurance studies in specific settings can all contribute important data. Such data can document which approaches and techniques are efficacious and which are not; when intervention can be the most effective in cost and outcome; what occupational therapy can contribute to maintenance of functional gains after discharge; and how occupational therapy can improve productivity without sacrificing positive functional outcomes for individual patients.

# REFERENCES

1. Bell E, Jurek K, Wilson T: Hand skill measurement: A gauge for treatment. *Am J Occup Ther* 30:80-86,1976
2. Warren M: Relationship of constructional apraxia and body scheme disorders to dressing performance in adult CVA. *Am J Occup Ther* 35:431-437, 1981
3. Diller L, Buxbaum J, Chiotelis S: Relearning motor skills in hemiplegia: Error analysis. *Genet Psychol Monographs* 85:249-286, 1972
4. Charait SE: A comparison of volar and dorsal splinting of the hemiplegic hand. *Am J Occup Ther* 22:319-321, 1968
5. Snook JH: Spasticity reduction splint. *Am J Occup Ther* 33: 648-651, 1979
6. Bryant NH, Candland L, Loewenstein R: Comparison of care and cost outcomes for stroke patients with and without home care. *Stroke* 5:54-59, 1974
7. Lehmann JF, DeLateur BJ, Fowler RS Jr, Warren CG, Arnhold R, Schertzer G, Hurka R, Whitmore JJ, Masock AJ, Chambers KH: Stroke: Does rehabilitation affect outcome? *Arch Phys Med Rehab* 56:375-382, 1975
8. Smith DS, Goldenberg E, Ashburn A, Kinsella G, Sheikh K, Brennan PJ, Meade TW, Zutshi DW, Perry JD, Reeback JS: Remedial therapy after stroke: A randomized controlled trial. *Br Med J* 282:517-520, 1981
9. Anderson TP, Baldridge M, Ettinger MG: Quality of care for completed stroke without rehabilitation: Evaluation by assessing patient outcomes. *Arch Phys Med Rehab* 60:103-107, 1979
10. Truscott BL, Kretschmann CM, Toole JF, Pajak TF: Early rehabilitative care in community hospitals: Effect on quality of survivorship following a stroke. *Stroke* 5:623-629, 1974

11. Garraway WM, Akhtar AJ, Prescott RJ, Hockey L: Management of acute stroke in the elderly: Preliminary results of a controlled trial. *Br Med J* 280:1040-1043, 1980
12. Smith ME, Garraway WM, Smith DL, Akhtar AJ: Therapy impact on functional outcome in a controlled trial of stroke rehabilitation. *Arch Phys Med Rehab* 63:21-24, 1982
13. Garraway WM, Akhtar AJ, Hockey L, Prescott RJ: Management of acute stroke in the elderly: Follow-up of a controlled trial. *Br Med J* 281:827-829, 1980

# THE EFFICACY OF REHABILITATION FOR STROKE PATIENTS

*Kenneth J. Ottenbacher, PhD, OTR, FAOTA*

## ABSTRACT

*The results of studies examining the effectiveness of rehabilitation therapy for patients who have suffered a cerebrovascular accident (CVA) are reviewed using recently developed quantitative methods that treat the literature review as a unique type of research. The results of the quantitative review indicate that patients receiving rehabilitation services performed at a higher level than patients in comparison or control conditions. Data analysis revealed that the average patient receiving rehabilitation services performed better than 58 percent of the patients in the comparison groups. In the contrasts that included a treatment group and a true control group that received no formal rehabilitation, the average patient in the treatment condition scored better than 63 percent of the patients in the control condition.*

*Although the reported treatment effects are in the range traditionally considered small, they have practical implications. Slight improvements in functional ability in patients who have suffered a CVA may make the difference between being institutionalized and remaining at home.*

*The results of the analysis indicate a significant relationship between the size of the treatment effect and the early initiation of rehabilitation services. The largest treatment effects were associated with the studies in which rehabilitation programming was begun soon after the onset of the CVA. In contrast, no significant relationship was found between the total amount or the duration of rehabilitation and the treatment effect size. Larger treatment effects were also associated with studies that included occupational therapy as part of the rehabilitation program.*

*Study results are discussed in relation to several design variables and study characteristics associated with patient performance. The limitations and the advantages of quantitative reviewing procedures are identified, and their potential usefulness in rehabilitation research is briefly discussed.*

## INTRODUCTION

The development and the implementation of rehabilitative programs for patients with functional deficits due to cerebrovascular accident (CVA) have progressed rapidly over the past decade. Trombly notes that people with CVA constitute the single largest diagnostic category treated by occupational therapists working with the adult population (1). Despite the widespread application of therapeutic rehabilitation with these patients, there is little consensus regarding the efficacy of the rehabilitative programs employed. For example, Lehmann et al. conducted a study in which a significant improvement in functional ability was attributed to a rehabilitation program (2). The results revealed gains in independence for six of seven activities-of-daily-living (ADL) categories. On the basis of these results Lehmann et al. argue that rehabilitation programs for CVA patients are effective and that no patient with hemiplegia should be denied the opportunity to receive treatment.

On the other hand, Feldman et al. conducted a randomized clinical trial of a comprehensive rehabilitation program (3). The treatment group received a program of intensive rehabilitation services while the control or comparison patients received standard functionally oriented medical care. Both the treatment group and the comparison group exhibited an increase in ADL independence over the period of the study, but there was no significant difference in their performance. Feldman et al. conclude, "The results suggest that the great majority of hemiparetic stroke victims can be rehabilitated adequately on medical and neurological wards without formal rehabilitation services if proper attention is given to ambulation and self-care activities" (3, p 306).

Unfortunately, traditional narrative attempts to interpret the accumulated research literature in this area have not resulted in any degree of empirical consensus. Lind has recently observed that only a handful of studies exist purporting to analyze the effects of rehabilitation on stroke patients and that "the results of these studies conflict and the conclusions vary widely" (4, p 133). In an attempt to bring more rigor and a degree of consensus to the research literature addressing the effectiveness of stroke rehabilitation programs, Lind synthesized the results of what he considered seven of the best available studies on rehabilitation outcome. The studies reviewed were analyzed according to the type of design employed, with particular attention to the ability of the design to control for selected threats to internal validity. Lind was particulary interested in assessing how well the seven studies controlled for the influence of maturation or selection-maturation effects as threats to internal validity. Lind cogently argues that these threats are a problem in research with stroke patients because of the possibility of spontaneous recovery. He states that "change which occurs naturally over time is referred to as a maturation effect, while the combined effects of biased sample selection and the maturation effect produce a selection-maturation interaction. Spontaneous recovery is an example of the maturation effect" (4, p 134).

From his analysis of the seven studies, Lind concludes,

The most prominent finding of this synthesis is that most of the improvement in functional ability is the result of spontaneous recovery. The inference which may be drawn is that there is limited potential for the rehabilitation of stroke patients beyond the improved functioning which may be expected to result from spontaneous recovery. (4, p 149)

Lind has made the assumption that if a study does not meet certain criteria related to research "quality," the results of the study are suspect (4). This assertion is credible when one is discussing a single investigation; however, the logic does not apply to a group of studies. Glass and his associates have correctly stated,

Research design has a logic of its own, but it is not a logic appropriate to research integration. The researcher does not want to perform a study deficient in some aspect of measurement or analysis, but it hardly follows that after a less-than-perfect study has been done, its findings should not be considered. A logic of research integration could lead to a description of design and analysis features and study of their covariance with research findings. If, for example, the covariance is quite small between the size of an experimental effect and whether or not subjects were volunteers, then the force of the criticism that some experiments used volunteers is clearly diminished. (5, pp 220-221).

The investigators involved in many primary research studies dealing with rehabilitation of stroke patients recommend further research on the specific hypothesis under study with the implied purpose of corroborating or contradicting reported findings. This call for additional research is based on the belief that empirical knowledge in the rehabilitation sciences should be cumulative. Evidence from multiple studies can be accumulated constructively and used effectively by policy makers, researchers, clinicians, and administrators only when it is synthesized systematically and logically. Narrative reviews of aggregated research literature have traditionally been used to achieve the goal of synthesizing information contained in multiple studies. The subjective and judgmental nature of some traditional literature reviews is unfortunate because integrative reviews are often influential in establishing or refuting the empirical legitimacy of a research finding.

The present study employed quantitative reviewing procedures to synthesize the evidence regarding the effectiveness of rehabilitation services for patients who have suffered a CVA. Techniques that sensitively integrate quantitative evidence have recently been developed and refined (5). These procedures treat the literature review as a unique type of research that requires the same rigorous methodology demanded of primary researchers (6). The methods enable the reviewer quantitatively to aggregate a large number of research studies and to make consensual judgments based on the results (6, 7). The procedures also allow systematic investigation of the effects of variation in study methodologies on study results, including the effects of differences in research design (5). It is hoped that the application of these procedures to evaluate the effectiveness of stroke rehabilitation programs will produce some insights that have eluded past reviews based on traditional narrative methods.

# METHODS

Eighty-eight reports that were broadly construed as potentially relevant to the topic of outcomes of stroke rehabilitation were supplied by the American Occupational Therapy Association as part of the Efficacy Data Project. The methods used to obtain the reports are described in the Introduction to this book. An independent computerized search by the author yielded two additional reports.

## CRITERIA FOR DETERMINING RELEVANCE

The reports were then judged for relevance on several specific criteria. The first criterion was that a study had to investigate the effects of a program of rehabilitation. To qualify as a rehabilitation program, the intervention had to include a set of procedures or treatment activities designed to improve the performance or the functional ability of people who had suffered a CVA.

The second criterion related to the subjects of the study. To be included in the review, the report had to include subjects whose primary medical diagnosis was hemiplegia or hemiparesis secondary to a CVA. Studies that included participants whose primary diagnosis was head trauma, brain tumor, or other nonstroke conditions were not included.

The third criterion for inclusion in the review was related to the type of dependent variable(s) employed in the report. One advantage of quantitative reviewing methods is that they permit the use of broad dependent variables. The use of multiple outcome measures provides a mechanism for evaluating the effects of multiple operationalism in a particular literature. Multiple operationalism may be generally defined as the use of many measures that share a similar theoretical concept or construct but employ different methods and procedures to assess that construct. For example, a given study investigating the efficacy of rehabilitation services for stroke patients may employ the Barthel Index as a measure of improvement in ADL. The argument could be made that the Barthel Index is a narrow measure and not representative of actual ADL abilities. If a second study employing similar treatment procedures but a totally different method of measuring ADL also reports improvements in this area, the argument that the rehabilitation treatment improves ADL in a broad or general sense is strengthened. Cooper notes that multiple operationalism has positive consequences because once a variable has been confirmed by two or more distinct measurement procedures, the uncertainty of its interpretation is greatly reduced (8).

The purpose of the present study was to evaluate the literature investigating the therapeutic effectiveness of rehabilitation services for stroke patients. Improvement or enhancement of functional abilities was broadly defined by performance on any measure of (a) motor or reflex functions, (b) cognitive or language abilities, (c) activities-of-daily-living skills, or (d) overall performance ability. A measure that could not be classified into one of the above groups was placed in a category labeled other. This category included outcome measures that did not occur with sufficient frequency to justify a separate category, for example, the setting to which a patient was discharged, vocational status, and the degree of bowel and bladder control

The final two criteria for inclusion in the review were related to a study's design and method of analysis. A study had to report a comparison between at least two groups or conditions. In the majority of cases the comparison was between a treatment group that received a comprehensive rehabilitation program and a comparison group that was provided standard medical care. For example, in the study by Feldman et al. (3) referred to previously, patients were randomly selected to determine whether they would receive the full range of rehabilitation services available or whether they would receive standard care on a medical or neurological ward. Patients in the treatment group received an individualized program of rehabilitation carried out by Department of Physical Medicine and Rehabilitation personnel. Patients on the medical or neurological wards (the comparison group) received a program of functionally oriented medical care supervised by the personnel of the wards. In some cases a within-subject design was used; the comparison or control condition comprised patients who later served as the experimental group.

Finally, a study had to report findings and results in a manner that allowed quantitative analysis. That is, a report had to include quantitative data related to the outcome of the comparisons, such as $t$ or $F$ ratios, means, standard deviations, and $p$ levels, in sufficient detail that the appropriate measure of effect size could be computed (the next section discusses measures of effect size).

With the general boundaries of the review determined, the next step was to identify aspects of the studies that might be related to study outcomes. These variables fell into four general categories. The first category was subject characteristics, including information on the number of subjects used in the study and their mean age. In addition, information related to sex, educational and socioeconomic status, and the number of patients who were identifed as right hemiplegics, left hemiplegics, or bilateral hemiplegics was recorded when available in the report. The second category included information related to the independent and dependent variables and the design characteristics of the study, such as (a) whether the design was preexperimental, quasi-experimental, or true experimental, (b) whether it was between subjects or within subjects, (c) what type of assignment was used (i.e., random, matching, or preexisting groups), (d) whether the outcome measure was blindly recorded, (e) how much time elapsed between the study's initiation and the measurement, (f) whether the outcome measure was standardized or informal, and (g) whether occupational therapy was included as part of the rehabilitation program. The third category of study characteristics included aspects of the study's outcome such as (a) the statistical test used, (b) the test value reported, (c) the accompanying probability level, and (d) the degree of freedom associated with error. The final category, labeled retrieval characteristics, included the year of publication and the source of publication, including whether the study was conducted inside or outside the United States. Figures 1 and 2 are the coding forms that were used.

The foregoing information was coded for all of the studies meeting the previously outlined criteria. It was then subjected to further analysis.

## QUANTIFYING STUDY OUTCOMES

Glass (9) and Cohen (10) have popularized procedures capable of uncovering systematic variation in study results. These procedures involve the calculation of a study's effect sizes and the analysis of these effect sizes in relation to study and design characteristics. Cohen defines an effect size as "the degree to which the null hypothesis is false" (10, pp 9-10).

Figure 1

## GENERAL EVALUATION FORM

ID_____

Authors_____

_____

Title    _____

_____

Source  _____

_____

Subjects

   Total number_____ Age_____Male_____ Female_____

   Left hemiplegics_____Right hemiplegics_____

   Length post stroke_____Length of study_____

Location of Study

   Major urban hospital_____

   University research hospital_____

   General hospital_____

   Rehabilitation center_____

   Other_____

General Design

   Group comparison (between subjects)_____

   Group comparison (within subjects)_____

   Correlational_____

Subject Assignment

   Random_____ Matching_____

   Combination (random and matching)_____

   Preexisting groups_____ Other_____

Comments

Figure 2

## GROUP COMPARISON

ID _____

Complete one of these for each comparison (hypothesis test) in the study.

Outcome Measure (specific test if available)

Motor/reflex_____

Language_____

Visual perceptual_____

Social_____

Self-help (ADL)_____

Vocational_____

Other_____

Measure standardized   Yes_____   No_____   Can't Tell_____

Measure blindly recorded   Yes_____   No_____   Can't Tell_____

Type of Design

Preexperimental_____ Quasi-experimental_____

Time-series_____ True experimental_____

Other_____

Outcome

Test value_____                    $p$ value_____

Effect size_____

Effect size from primary data   Yes_____   No_____

Type of Treatment _____

Include OT  Yes___ No___

Treatment Program Administered by   Family_____   Therapist_____

Nurse_____   Trainer_____   MD_____   Team_____

Other_____

Multiple Degrees-of-Freedom Study   Yes_____   No_____

Measures of effect size that are appropriate for use with a wide variety of research designs and analytic procedures have been presented by Cohen (10). The primary measure of effect size employed in this investigation, referred to as the $d$ index, is used to evaluate the statistical comparison between two groups. One of the criteria for inclusion in the review was that a two-group comparison be made in a study. Of the ninety potentially relevant studies originally retrieved for the review, sixty-eight did not meet at least one of the criteria presented in the previous section. Twenty-two studies remained for inclusion in the quantitative review. Unfortunately, eight of them were based on data from one sample only, so they were eliminated. That left fourteen studies, which are identified at the end of this chapter.

Several of the fourteen studies included in the review contained more than one comparison between two groups. For example, Feigenson et al. (11) conducted an investigation comparing the performance of patients in stroke and nonstroke units. Four outcome measures were employed, including discharge placement, ambulation status at discharge, independence in ADL, and length of stay at the rehabilitation facility. Thus, multiple comparisons were made based on different dependent measures employed within a single study. Together, the fourteen studies contained a total of fifty hypothesis tests for two-group comparisons evaluating the effectiveness of rehabilitation programs for patients who had suffered a CVA.

As noted above, the measure of effect size computed for each two-group comparison was the $d$ index. The $d$ index gauges the difference between the means of two groups in terms of their common (average) standard deviation. If $d = .30$, it indicates that .30 of a standard deviation separates the two sample means. Cohen (10) has defined a $d$ index of .20 to .50 as a small effect size, .50 to .80 as a medium one, and greater than .80 as a large one. This classification system may not have much intuitive appeal. For this reason Cohen also presents a percentage of distribution overlap measure called $U_3$. This measure indicates what percentage of the population with the smaller mean is exceeded by 50 percent of the population with the larger mean. The $U_3$ value for a $d$ index of .30 is 61.8. This value means that the average person in the group with the larger mean (usually the treatment group) has a "score" greater than approximately 62 percent of the individuals in the group with the lower mean. A table for converting the $d$ index to $U_3$ is presented by Cohen (10, p 22).

Friedman (12) has presented formulas for computing $d$ index estimates from traditional inferential statistical values such as $t$

and $F$ ratios. For example, the formula for converting a $t$ value to a $d$ index is as follows:

$$d = \frac{2(t)}{\sqrt{\text{df error}}}$$

where $t$ equals the value of the $t$ test for the associated comparison and df error equals the degrees of freedom associated with the error term of the $t$ test. In cases in which the inferential statistical values were not reported, an estimated index of effect size was computed from significance levels and sample sizes. In addition, Glass (9) has described procedures for computing effect sizes in situations where nonparametric statistics or some form of descriptive statistics such as percentages is used.

Finally, Hedges (13) has demonstrated that $d$ indexes may be biased as the sample size becomes smaller (i.e., fewer than fifty). Therefore, Hedges's correction factors were employed in this investigation to adjust for potentially inflated effect sizes from small samples ( < 50). When a study reported a nonsignificant result but not enough information was provided to determine an effect size, an effect size of 0.00 was assumed.

## RESULTS

A total of 2,362 subjects participated in the fourteen studies (fifty hypothesis tests). Approximately 51 percent of the subjects were males, 49 percent females. Slightly more patients were diagnosed as right hemiplegics or hemiparetics (47 percent) than left hemiplegics or hemiparetics (41 percent). The remaining 12 percent were diagnosed as bilateral or undifferentiated.

The mean age of participants was 65.2 years (SD = 6.35). Mean ages were generally reported for subjects at the beginning of the study. For those studies reporting ages at both the beginning and the end of the investigation, only the initial ages were included in determining the overall mean age across the studies. The mean year of report appearance was 1977 (SD = 4.38), and the mean length of time between the occurrence of the CVA and the onset of rehabilitation treatment was seven weeks.

The mean $d$ index for the fifty hypothesis tests was .20 (SD = .21). The $d$ indexes for all the hypothesis tests included in the review are displayed in Table 1. Each $d$ index is indicated by a combination of "stem" and "leaf" following the system of data presentation suggested by Tukey (14). The stem is the initial or beginning value of the $d$ index. It appears in the left-hand column of the table. The leaf values represent individual numbers, each of which is associated with the corresponding stem. For example, the numbers 6 and 7 (leaf) to the right of .5 (stem) in Table 1 represent $d$ indexes of .56 and .57 respectively. The stem and the leaf provide all the information of a histogram but also show the actual values of all $d$ indexes. Below the stem and leaf plot are the minimum and maximum $d$ indexes, along with the first- and third-quartile ($Q_1$, $Q_3$) means, the median, and the standard deviation.

Table 1
Stem and Leaf Plot Displaying $d$ Indexes from Studies Investigating the Efficacy of Rehabilitation for Patients with CVA

| Stem | Leaf | Total |
|------|------|-------|
| .9 | | |
| .8 | 6 | 1 |
| .7 | 6 | 1 |
| .6 | | |
| .5 | 67 | 2 |
| .4 | 39 | 2 |
| .3 | 013333359 | 9 |
| .2 | 022354 | 6 |
| .1 | 0111233455555678 | 16 |
| .0 | 00000222889 | 11 |
| -.1 | 6 | 1 |
| -.2 | 7 | 1 |

| | | | |
|---|---|---|---|
| Mean .20 | $Q_1$ .09 | Minimum -.27 |
| Median .15 | $Q_3$ .33 | Maximum .86 |
| Standard deviation .21 | | |

The U₃ value associated with a *d* index of .20 is 57.9. This means that the average performance of patients in the group or the condition receiving some form of rehabilitation service was better than 57.9 percent of the patients in control or comparison groups not receiving that service. Figure 3 presents a graphic display of the distributions of effect size for subjects receiving some form of rehabilitation service and those in the comparison or control groups. The distributions in Figure 3 are based on the assumption of normally distributed effect sizes for the population of studies. To the degree that this is a valid assumption, Figure 3 provides a useful heuristic device for comparing the performance of the treatment and comparison groups.

Hedges (15) has pointed out that the results of studies and associated effect sizes will vary based on chance. That is, because researchers take samples from populations, the means of the samples will not always be identical to the population mean nor to other sample estimates. The amount of variability in sample means taken from a single population is a function of the number of data points on which the sample means are based. The possibility therefore exists that considerable variance may occur within a collection of effect sizes because of sampling error. Hedges (15) and Rosenthal and Rubin (16) have proposed the use

Figure 3
Normal Curves Illustrating the Effect of Rehabilitation Received by the Treatment Groups in Relation to the Control or Comparison Groups

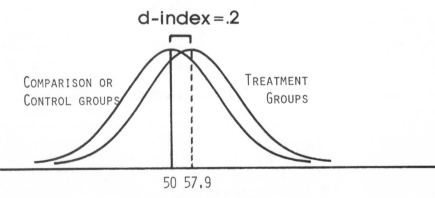

of a homogeneity analysis to test whether the variance exhibited in a set of effect sizes is explainable by sampling error. If the homogeneity analysis reveals that the variance in the effect sizes is greater than expected by chance, the investigator may begin to examine other sources of variance due to study characteristics or design variables. The overall-homogeneity statistic ($H_T$) described by Hedges (15) was computed for the set of effect sizes ($d$ indexes). It indicated that the amount of variability in the collection of effect sizes exceeded that which would have been expected by chance. As a result, an analysis of effect sizes by specific design characteristics was considered justified.

## DESIGN CHARACTERISTICS AND EFFECT SIZE

As noted in the methods section, each study was coded on several characteristics related to study design. Individual studies were coded by the type of research design, based on criteria originally developed and presented by Campbell and Stanley (17). Designs were classified as preexperimental, quasi-experimental, or true experimental. Preexperimental designs included one-group pretest-posttest designs or variations in which one group was originally evaluated, provided intervention, and tested again to determine the effects of intervention. The quasi-experimental design category included a variety of designs with several similar characteristics. Generally, subject groups rather than individuals were assigned to intervention and nonintervention conditions. The final category included true experimental designs, employing a traditional pretest-posttest control-group design with a random assignment of the subjects or a combination of random assignment and matching of individual subjects.

Two PhD-trained evaluators rated each study design according to the above design categories. An overall agreement index of 91 percent was obtained for labeling the designs employed in the fourteen studies included in the review. The mean $d$ index associated with each type of experimental design, along with related descriptive information, appears in Table 2. An inspection of Table 2 reveals that the largest mean effect size was associated with designs classified as preexperimental. The mean $d$ indexes for comparisons associated with quasi-experimental and true experimental designs were somewhat smaller.

The $d$ indexes employed in this study are based on comparisons that are not independent from one another; that is, more than one comparison ($d$ index) was obtained from some studies. Therefore, using inferential statistics to test whether effect sizes differed significantly across design categories may not be warranted (8, 18). In the manner of Smith (19) an informal criterion was adopted by which $d$ indexes were considered to differ reliably from one another if they were more than two standard errors apart. Presenting the standard error of the mean for effects provides an easy-to-interpret measure of difference for the means of various conditions. For example, the mean effect size for true experimental designs was .17, with a standard error of .05 (see Table 2). Effect sizes ranging from +2 standard errors (.27) to -2 standard errors (.07) would not be considered reliably different from the mean effect size for true experimental designs. The use of this convention produced no reliable difference among mean effect sizes across the types of research designs evident in the fifty $d$ indexes computed from the studies that were reviewed.

Effect sizes were also analyzed according to the procedures for assigning subjects. For the fifteen comparisons employing random assignment, the mean $d$ index was .23; for the twelve contrasts using matching or some combination of matching and randomization, it was .19. Convenience samples or preexisting groups were employed in twenty-three of the comparisons and were also associated with a mean $d$ index of .19. Across the types of procedures for assigning subjects, no reliable difference existed on the previously described criterion of two standard errors.

## THE INDEPENDENT VARIABLE
## AND EFFECT SIZE

The independent variable, the treatment of particular interest in this study, was the effectiveness of rehabilitation procedures.

Table 2
Descriptive Information for $d$ Indexes Associated with Different Research Designs

| Design | $N$ | Mean | SD[a] | SEM[b] | $U_3$ |
|---|---|---|---|---|---|
| Preexperimental | 10 | .25 | .19 | .06 | 60% |
| Quasi-experimental | 23 | .21 | .20 | .04 | 58% |
| True experimental | 17 | .17 | .18 | .05 | 57% |

[a]SD = Standard deviation
[b]SEM = Standard error of the mean

Rehabilitation procedures were broadly defined as services "concerned with the restoration and development of physiological and psychological function in order to improve performance and behavior" (20, p 176). These services were often provided by a variety of rehabilitation personnel, including rehabilitation nurses, occupational therapists, physical therapists, speech pathologists, rehabilitation counselors, psychologists, and others.

Of particular interest in this investigation was the impact of occupational therapy on the effectiveness of rehabilitation services for stroke patients. Smith, Garraway, Smith, and Akhtar, in their study of rehabilitation outcomes (21), demonstrated that the early presence of occupational therapy services was positively associated with improved patient performance. To investigate the relationship of occupational therapy to outcomes with patients, studies were coded for the presence or the absence of occupational therapy in the rehabilitation program provided to patients. In thirty-five of the comparisons, occupational therapy was a component of the rehabilitation program. The mean $d$ index for these comparisons was .22. Occupational therapy was not included in the rehabilitation programs associated with twelve comparisons. Their mean $d$ index was .17. In three comparisons it was not possible to determine occupational therapy's involvement. The mean $d$ index for these three was .15.

If the twelve comparisons associated with no occupational therapy are combined with the three in which no determination of occupational therapy involvement could be made, a reliable difference between the mean effect sizes exists. The comparisons associated with occupational therapy show a mean effect size reliably larger than the comparisons not associated with occupational therapy do, using the convention of two standard errors.

## DEPENDENT VARIABLES AND EFFECT SIZE

As noted previously, the outcome measures were categorized as motor/reflex, activities of daily living, cognitive/language, overall functional assessments, and other. The mean $d$ indexes and related descriptive data for each of the categories of dependent measures appear in Table 3. Inspection of the information in Table 3 reveals that dependent measures classified as activities of daily living (ADL) were associated with the largest mean $d$ index. These measures were also the most frequently encountered type of dependent measure. In general, this analysis indicates that improvement in a variety of outcome measures was relatively even across the multiple comparisons. The application of the two-standard-error criterion revealed no reliable differences among any of the outcome measures, although more improvement was generally seen in motor/reflex and ADL measures than in cognitive/language measures (see Table 3).

A related analysis explored the association beween $d$ indexes and the use of a standardized or informal dependent measure. Standardized measures were those developed for a specific population, administered in a prescribed manner, and providing a standardized score. The Barthel Index and the Klein-Bell Assessment represented examples of standardized measures. Other more informal assessments were frequently developed by the authors for a particular study and relied on comparisons between subjects in the specific study or clinical judgments of the investigators. The mean $d$ index for the seventeen comparisons associated with standardized measures was .18, whereas the mean $d$ index for the twenty-eight comparisons based on informal measures was .22. It was not possible to determine whether the outcome measure was standardized or informal in five of the comparisons. The mean $d$ index for these five comparisons was .19. No reliable difference existed across the fifty effect sizes based on whether the outcome measure was standardized or informal.

Data concerning how the dependent measure was recorded

Table 3
Descriptive Information for $d$ Indexes According to Type of Dependent Measure

| Dependent Measure | $N$ | Mean | SD[a] | SEM[b] | $U_3$ |
|---|---|---|---|---|---|
| Motor/reflex | 13 | .22 | .26 | .07 | 59% |
| Cognitive/language | 5 | .14 | .12 | .05 | 56% |
| ADL | 15 | .24 | .25 | .07 | 60% |
| Overall function | 8 | .15 | .13 | .05 | 56% |
| Other | 9 | .20 | .19 | .06 | 58% |

[a]SD = Standard deviation
[b]SEM = Standard error of the mean

were also coded and included in the analysis. The dependent measure was blindly recorded in eight of the comparisons, and these were associated with a mean $d$ index of .47. For the remaining forty-two comparisons, in which the dependent measure was not blindly recorded or there was not enough information to determine how the dependent measure was recorded, the mean $d$ index was .15. The two-standard-error assessment indicated that the difference between the mean $d$ indexes for whether or not the dependent measure was blindly recorded was reliably different.

## MISCELLANEOUS ANALYSES

The data on effect size were analyzed according to whether the study had been conducted inside or outside the United States. The results revealed a mean $d$ index of .18 for comparisons derived from studies in the United States versus a mean $d$ index of .24 for comparisons obtained from studies outside. This analysis suggests that the studies outside the United States generally reported larger treatment effects than the studies inside did. The difference in mean $d$ indexes was not reliably different using the two-standard-error convention.

Correlations were computed between the year a report appeared and the $d$ index ($r = .03, p = NS$); the number of subjects per study and the effect size ($r = .13, p = NS$); the average age of subjects in the study and the effect size ($r = -.52, p < .05$); and the average lapse of time between the occurrence of the CVA and the entrance into a rehabilitation program, and the effect size ($r = -.32, p < .05$). The last two significant correlations suggest that larger effect sizes ($d$ indexes) were inversely related to the patient's age and the amount of time that elapsed beween CVA and the beginning of the rehabilitation program. The correlation between the total duration of the treatment (the rehabilitation program) and the $d$ index was not significant ($r = .11, p = NS$).

## DISCUSSION

The effectiveness of rehabilitation programs for patients with hemiplegia of hemiparesis is currently an issue generating considerable professional debate (4, 22). In the present political and economic climate the cost effectiveness and the therapeutic impact of many rehabilitation services will continue to be questioned until a more empirically convincing data base can be generated supporting rehabilitation outcomes.

## THE EFFECTS OF TREATMENT: CAUSES AND CORRELATIONS

The reviewing techniques employed in this investigation have demonstrated that rehabilitation programs for stroke patients do produce quantifiable effects. The overall mean effect size reported for the studies reviewed was .20. This effect size was associated with a $U_3$ value of 57.9, suggesting that the average subject in the treatment condition receiving rehabilitation performed better than approximately 58 percent of the subjects in the comparison condition. The overall mean effect of .20 was in the range Cohen considers a small treatment effect (10). This does not mean, however, that the therapeutic implications of the overall mean effect are small. Rosenthal and Rubin (23) have introduced the binomial effect size display (BESD) to help interpret the values of effect size. The BESD answers the question, What is the effect on the success rate of a treatment procedure? The BESD presents the change in success rate attributable to a treatment. For a $d$ index of .20 the BESD is equal to 10 percent or, for example, a change in success rate from 40 to 50 percent. The use of the BESD to demonstrate an increase in performance or success rate due to treatment more clearly communicates the real-world importance of the treatment effects than do the commonly used effect-size estimators based on the proportion of variance accounted for by the independent variable (23). The importance of the treatment effect is enhanced when one considers that in the great majority of the two-group comparisons, the comparison being made was between one group receiving some standard treatment or rehabilitation (the comparison group) and another group receiving more intensive or specialized rehabilitation (the treatment group).

In nine comparisons an evaluation was made between a group receiving rehabilitation services and a true control group that did not receive rehabilitation services. For example, in the study by Smith et al. (24) patients were randomly assigned to a group that received intensive rehabilitation, a group that received conventional rehabilitation, or a group that received no routine rehabilitation services (24). Comparisons such as this provide a more direct test of the efficacy of rehabilitation programs for stroke patients. The mean $d$ index for the nine comparisons between a treatment group and a control group was .33. The BESD for these comparisons was .16, indicating a success rate of 16 percent. Even though this effect size is still in the range Cohen considers small, the effect has obvious therapeutic implications. Small effects may not often be associated with statistical significance; therefore, negative conclusions regarding the efficacy of rehabilitation may be drawn from an individual study, particularly from those with small sample sizes. Friedman et al. (25) have elaborated on the dangers inherent in equating statistical significance with practical significance in clinical research, in which treatment effects are difficult to isolate and measure. Lind (4) acknowledges this fact in his review of rehabilitation studies with stroke patients. He observes, "Improvements which are attributable to comprehensive rehabilitation programs are so slight as to escape reliable measurement. However, improvements in functional ability may occur and may, in some cases, make the critical difference between being institutionalized or being at home" (p 148). The results of this investigation lend quantitative support to Lind's conclusion.

The suggestion that design characteristics are an important consideration in evaluating the results of rehabilitation efficacy studies for stroke patients was only partially supported. No reliable difference between effect sizes was found across the types of design or the procedures for subject assignment. A reliable difference between mean effect sizes was found based on how the dependent measure was recorded. The designs in which the outcome measure was blindly recorded were associated with a larger mean effect size than those in comparisons that did not blindly evaluate patient performance.

Some authorities in rehabilitation medicine have questioned the empirical validity of rehabilitation for stroke patients based on the weakness of study designs (4). The implication is that poorly controlled or poorly designed studies may produce significant results in favor of the intervention that would not appear in more rigorously controlled investigations. The results of the present study did not support this contention. The possibility exists that design factors produce results in the opposite directions. For example, the argument could be made that the larger variances commonly associated with or attributed to poorly controlled or designed studies may contribute "noise" that masks the perception or the evidence of a successful outcome. This argument is partially supported in the present study by the finding that comparisons associated with studies in which the outcome measure was blindly recorded produced larger effects, on the average, than studies in which the dependent measure was not blindly recorded. Clearly the issue of how study design variables influence study outcomes in a particular body of research literature is an empirical question best answered through the application of quantitative reviewing procedures.

The fact that studies including occupational therapy services were associated with a larger mean effect size than studies that did not include occupational therapy certainly indicates an area in need of further investigation. This is particularly true in view of the study by Smith et al. (21) referred to previously, in which the early presence of occupational therapy services was associated with positive patient outcomes. It is important to qualify this finding by noting that the relationship is associational in nature; no causal inference can be drawn between the presence of occupational therapy and improved performance.

Another interesting finding relates to the correlation between effect size and patient age. A significant negative correlation was found between age and $d$ indexes across the fifty comparisons. This correlation suggests that larger treatment effects were associated with younger patients, smaller effects with older patients. Again, this finding is associational not causal in nature and may be due to a third factor not included in the analysis. For example, Lehmann et al. (2) report that older patients were more likely to have the most severe strokes and that the severity of the CVA may be the variable influencing the outcome. When the severity of the stroke was controlled for in the Lehmann et al. study, the correlation between age and patient outcome was reduced considerably. Unfortunately the majority of the studies included in this review did not provide information on the severity of the CVA so this variable could not be included in the analysis.

The duration of the rehabilitation programs provided in the reviewed studies was not associated with improved performance as measured by effect size. However, a significant relationship was found between the size of the effect and the length of time after the CVA until rehabilitation was initiated. The largest effect sizes were associated with the studies in which rehabilitation programming was begun relatively early. This result provides support for the early initiation of rehabilitation procedures for stroke patients and corroborates the findings of Smith et al. (21), who report that "early introduction of rehabilitation by therapists may be more important than the amount or duration of the treatment" (p 21).

## LIMITATIONS

The ability of quantitative reviewing procedures to test or evaluate certain relationships among aggregated studies does not mean that all problems of conceptualization or methodological artifact can be resolved. Alternative conceptualizations may rival those based on multiple studies in the same manner that alternative conceptualizations may account for the results of a particular primary investigation. In addition, certain factors important to intervention outcomes cannot easily be assessed across many primary studies. For example, the intensity or the integrity of the treatment program is often difficult or impossible to evaluate across studies. An investigation may contain a very convincing operational definition of the intervention strategy but provide little information concerning how effectively the treatment program was actually implemented. Issues related to the strength and the integrity of intervention programs may have an influence on treatment outcomes that both traditional reviewing procedures and quantitative reviewing methods are unable to evaluate.

Some readers may feel that quantitative reviewing procedures can create an illusion of statistical objectivity that is not justified by the data obtained from the review (26). In terms of the specific statistical procedures employed, the fact that statistical tests of several hypotheses may be included in a single study suggests that estimates of effect size based on those statistical tests are not independent data points. This introduces the problem of nonindependence into the analysis and may result in inflated or unreliable estimates if inferential statistical procedures are used to analyze the data. The role of inferential statistical procedures in the data analysis stage of quantitative reviewing is controversial, and for this reason the data on effect size in this study (the $d$ indexes) were analyzed descriptively.

Another potential limitation of the present review is the issue of missing data. The authors of the reviewed studies did not report all of the possible statistical information from which an effect size can be calculated. Hence it was not always possible to derive all the potential effect sizes for a given study. Several studies included in this review failed to report one or more sets of results in sufficient detail to compute or estimate an effect size. Some studies were more defective than others in not reporting important information. Other reviewers have encountered this problem of missing data and commented on its possible effects (5, 8). For example, Cooper (8) argues that there may be a systematic bias in the types of data that are missing from studies. Authors may be less likely to report specific data from analyses yielding nonsignificant results for comparisons between groups and conditions. To the extent that investigators fail to report results of nonsignificant outcomes, a degree of systematic bias is introduced into the reporting of study findings. That problem was dealt with in this investigation by assigning an effect size of 0.00 to any nonsignificant comparison for which data were not provided in the primary study. This is a conservative correction, and its application requires the author to state that a nonsignificant test was conducted.

In spite of the above limitations the quantitative reviewing procedures applied in this study represent a significant advance over traditional narrative attempts to integrate a body of research literature. As Rosenthal has noted, the "procedures are not perfect, we can use them inappropriately, and we will make mistakes. Nevertheless, the alternative to the systematic, explicit, quantitative procedures is even less perfect, even more likely to be applied inappropriately, and even more likely to lead us to error" (18, p 17).

The results of this investigation have demonstrated that treatment effects from rehabilitation programs designed for stroke patients are evident if the proper techniques are employed to identify them. The overall mean effect size associated with rehabilitative services is small, and additional questions remain to be answered regarding the efficacy of rehabilitation programs for stroke patients. These questions include the following: For whom does rehabilitation work best? Are certain programs better for certain patients? When should patients be enrolled to achieve maximum benefit? How long do the effects of treatment last? These important questions need to be addressed by researchers in the rehabilitation specialties. Professional service providers, including occupational therapy personnel, cannot and should not wait for the one study that will resolve these issues. The results of this investigation demonstrate that the professional can begin to answer some of the questions if current studies and future research are properly synthesized.

# REFERENCES

1. Trombly CA: *Occupational Therapy for Physical Dysfunction*, ed 2. Baltimore: Williams & Wilkins, 1983
2. Lehmann JF, DeLateur BJ, Fowler RS Jr, Warren CG, Arnhold R, Schertzer G, Hurka R, Whitmore JJ, Masock AJ, Chambers KH: Stroke: Does rehabilitation affect outcome? *Arch Phys Med Rehab* 56:375-382, 1975
3. Feldman DJ, Lee PR, Unterecker J, Lloyd K, Rusk HA, Toole A: A comparison of functionally oriented medical care and formal rehabilitation in the management of patients with hemiplegia due to cerebrovascular disease. *J Chron Dis* 15:297-310, 1962
4. Lind K: A synthesis of studies on stroke rehabilitation. *J Chron Dis* 35:133-149, 1982
5. Glass GV, McGaw B, Smith ML: *Meta-Analysis in Social Research.* Beverly Hills, CA: Sage Publications, 1981
6. Cooper HM: Scientific guidelines for conducting integrative research reviews. *Rev Educ Res* 52:291-302, 1982
7. Light RJ, Pillemer DB: Numbers and narrative: Combining their strengths in research reviews. *Harvard Educ Rev* 52:1-26, 1982

8. Cooper HM: *The Integrative Research Review: A Social Science Approach.* Beverly Hills, CA: Sage Publications, 1984

9. Glass GV: Summarizing effect sizes. In *New Directions for Methodology of Social and Behavioral Science: Quantitative Assessment of Research Domains,* R. Rosenthal, Editor. San Francisco, CA: Jossey-Bass, 1980

10. Cohen, J: *Statistical Power Analysis for the Behavioral Sciences,* rev ed. New York: Academic Press, 1977

11. Feigenson JS, Gitlow HS, Greenberg SD: The disability oriented rehabilitation unit--A major factor in influencing stroke outcome. *Stroke* 10:5-8, 1979

12. Friedman H: Magnitude of experimental effect and a table for its rapid estimation. *Psychol Bull* 70:245-251, 1968

13. Hedges LV: Distribution theory for Glass's estimator of effect size and related estimators. *J Educ Stat* 6:107-128, 1981

14. Tukey JW: *Exploratory Data Analysis.* Reading, MA: Addison-Wesley, 1977

15. Hedges LV: A random effects model for effect sizes. *Psychol Bull* 93:388-395, 1983

16. Rosenthal R, Rubin DB: Comparing effect sizes of independent studies. *Psychol Bull* 92:500-504, 1982

17. Campbell DT, Stanley JC: *Experimental and Quasi-Experimental Designs for Research.* Chicago: Rand-McNally, 1966

18. Rosenthal R: *Meta-Analytic Procedures for Social Research.* Beverly Hills, CA: Sage Publications, 1984

19. Smith ML: Sex bias in counseling and psychotherapy. *Psychol Bull* 87:392-407, 1980

20. Anderson TP, Kottke FJ: Stroke rehabilitation: A reconsideration of some common attitudes. *Arch Phys Med Rehab* 59:175-181, 1978

21. Smith ME, Garraway WM, Smith DL, Akhtar AJ: Therapy impact on functional outcome in a controlled trial of stroke rehabilitation. *Arch Phys Med Rehab* 63:21-24, 1982

22. Feigenson JS: Stroke rehabilitation: Effectiveness, benefits, and cost. Some practical considerations (editorial). *Stroke* 10:1-4, 1979

23. Rosenthal R, Rubin DB: A simple, general purpose display of magnitude of experiment effect. *J Educ Psychol* 74:166-169, 1982

24. Smith DS, Goldenberg E, Ashburn A, Kinsella G, Sheikh K, Brennan PJ, Meade TW, Zutshi DW, Perry JD, Reeback JS: Remedial therapy after stroke: A randomized controlled trial. *Br Med J* 282:517-520, 1981

25. Freidman JA, Chalmer TC, Smith H, Kuebler RR: The importance of beta, the type II error and sample size in the design and interpretation of the randomized control trial. *New Eng J Med* 299:690-694, 1978
26. Cook TD, Leviton L: Reviewing the literature: A comparison of traditional methods with meta-analysis. *J Person* 48:449-472, 1980

## STUDIES INCLUDED IN THE QUANTITATIVE SYNTHESIS

Anderson TP, Baldridge M, Ettinger MG: Quality of care for completed stroke without rehabilitation: Evaluation by assessing patient outcomes. *Arch Phys Med Rehab* 60:103-107, 1979

Brocklehurst JC, Andrews K, Richards B, Laycock PJ: How much physical therapy for patients with stroke? *Br Med J* 279:1307-1310, 1978

Bryant NH, Candland L, Loewenstein R: Comparison of care and cost outcomes for stroke patients with and without home care. *Stroke* 5:54-59, 1974

Feigenson JS, Gitlow HS, Greenberg SD: The disability oriented rehabilitation unit--A major factor influencing stroke outcome. *Stroke* 10:5-8, 1979

Feldman DJ, Lee PR, Unterecker J, Lloyd K, Rusk HA, Toole A: A comparison of functionally oriented medical care and formal rehabilitation in the management of patients with hemiplegia due to cerebrovascular disease. *J Chron Dis* 15:297-310, 1962

Garraway WM, Akhtar AJ, Hockey L, Prescott RJ: Management of acute stroke in the elderly: Follow-up of a controlled trial. *Br Med J* 281:827-829, 1980

Inaba M, Edberg E, Montgomery J, Gillis MK: Effectiveness of functional training, active exercise, and resistive exercise for patients with hemiplegia. *Phys Ther* 53:28-35, 1973

Lehmann JF, DeLateur BJ, Fowler RS Jr, Warren CG, Arnhold R, Schertzer G, Hurka R, Whitmore JJ, Masock AJ, Chambers KH: Stroke: Does rehabilitation affect outcome? *Arch Phys Med Rehab* 56:375-382, 1975

McCann BC, Culbertson RA: Comparison of two systems for stroke rehabilitation in a general hospital. *J Am Geriatrics Soc* 24:211-216, 1976

Smith DS, Goldenberg E, Ashburn A, Kinsella G, Sheikh K, Brennan PJ, Meade TW, Zutshi DW, Perry JD, Reeback JS: Remedial therapy after stroke: A randomized controlled trial.

*Br Med J* 282:517-520, 1981

Smith ME, Garraway WM, Smith DL, Akhtar AJ: Therapy impact on functional outcome in a controlled trial of stroke rehabilitation. *Arch Phys Med Rehab* 63:21-24, 1982

Stern PH, McDowell F, Miller JM, Robinson M: Effects of facilitation exercise techniques in stroke rehabilitation: *Arch Phys Med Rehab* 51:526-531, 1970

Waylonis GW, Keith MW, Asseff JN: Stroke rehabilitation in a midwestern county. *Arch Phys Med Rehab* 54:151-155, 1973

Wood-Dauphinee S, Shapiro S, Bass E, Fletcher C, Georges P, Hansby V, Mendelsohn B: A randomized trial of team care following stroke. *Stroke* 15:864-872, 1984

# Appendix

# SUPPLEMENTARY BIBLIOGRAPHY, JANUARY 1983-JUNE 1985

*Kathy L. Kaplan, MS, OTR*

Health care personnel are aware how hard it is to find time to read relevant literature in the field. In the experience of the contributors to the Efficacy Data Project, even with large blocks of time specified for a literature review, identifying, retrieving, evaluating, and integrating research findings is a lengthy process. Just as clinicians must set priorities on how to spend their time most effectively, the staff of this project also had to establish boundaries on the collection process.

The original search was conducted in December 1982 at the National Library of Medicine. An updated search included some overlap of references from 1982, plus acquisitions through June 1985. The Medline computerized data base provided a list of titles, from which the most relevant were selected. Key words for the search parameters included *stroke, hemiplegia, evaluation studies, activities of daily living (ADL), rehabilitation, occupational therapy, efficacy,* and *outcome assessment.* Not all of the potentially relevant studies could be secured. Therefore, the key words were combined to yield the most promising citations. Relevant articles were retrieved and reviewed by project personnel, but were not sent to the panel for examination of the validity of the studies.

The articles reflect a broad perspective on the outcomes of stroke rehabilitation. Some pertain to the stroke recovery process, demographic features of patient subgroups, or predictive factors of outcome as related to rehabilitation in general. Others relate more directly to occupational therapy assessment and treatment, examining the effects of timeliness of referrals, length of stay, functional level, and outcome as measured by activities-of-daily-living skills. Clinicians may find the articles of benefit in--
- Enhancing their knowledge of the needs of stroke patients.
- Increasing their awareness of treatment effects.
- Improving the data base from which to justify new or existing programs.
- Expanding their familiarity with study designs that may be replicable or may stimulate further research.

## BIBLIOGRAPHY

Allen, CMC: Predicting the outcome of acute stroke: A prognostic score. *J Neurology, Neurosurgery, and Psychiatry* 47:475-480, 1984

Andrews K, Brocklehurst JC, Richards B, Laycock PJ: The recovery of the severely disabled stroke patient. *Rheumatology and Rehab* 21:225-230, 1982

Carter LT, Howard BE, O'Neil WA: Effectiveness of cognitive skill remediation in acute stroke patients. *Am J Occup Ther* 37:320-326, 1983

Dove HG, Schneider KC, Wallace JD: Evaluating and predicting outcome of acute cerebral vascular accident. *Stroke* 15:858-864, 1984

Garraway M: Stroke rehabilitation units: Concepts, evaluation, and unresolved issues. *Stroke* 16:178-181, 1985

Henley S, Pettit S, Todd-Pokropek A, Tupper A: Who goes home? Predictive factors in stroke recovery. *J Neurology, Neurosurgery, and Psychiatry* 48:1-6, 1985

Herman JM, Culpepper L, Franks P: Patterns of utilization, disposition, and length of stay among stroke patients in a community hospital setting. *J Am Geriatrics Soc* 32:421-426, 1984

Hertanu JS, Demopoulos JT, Yang WC, Calhoun WF, Fenigstein HA: Stroke rehabilitation: Correlation and prognostic value of computerized tomography and sequential functional assessments. *Arch Phys Med Rehab* 65:505-508, 1984

Holbrook M, Skilbeck CE: An activities index for use with stroke patients. *Age and Ageing* 12:166-170, 1983

Howard G, Till JS, Toole JF, Matthews C, Truscott BL: Factors influencing return to work following cerebral infarction. *JAMA* 253:226-232, 1985

Johnston MV, Keister M: Early rehabilitation for stroke patients: A new look. *Arch Phys Med Rehab* 65:437-441, 1984

Johnston MV, Keith RA: Cost-benefits of medical rehabilitation: Review and critique. *Arch Phys Med Rehab* 64:147-153, 1983

Kotila M, Waltimo O, Niemi ML, Laaksonen R, Lempinen M: The profile of recovery from stroke and factors influencing outcome. *Stroke* 15:1039-1044, 1984

Logigian MK, Samuels MA, Falconer J: Clinical exercise trial for stroke patients. *Arch Phys Med Rehab* 64:364-367, 1983

Marsh M: A day rehabilitation stroke program. *Arch Phys Med Rehab* 65:320-323, 1984

McClatchie G, Schuld W, Goodwin S: A maximized-ADL index of functional status for stroke patients. *Scand J Rehab Med* 15:155-163, 1983

Miller LS, Forer SK, Davis C: Rehabilitation social workers: Measuring their ability to predict discharge destination of rehabilitation patients. *Arch Phys Med Rehab* 65:87-88, 1984

Novack TA, Satterfield WT, Lyons K, Kolski G, Hackmeyer L, Connor M: Stroke onset and rehabilitation: Time lag as a factor in treatment outcome. *Arch Phys Med Rehab* 65:316-319, 1984

Reding M, Orto L, Willensky P, Fortuna I, Day N, Steiner SF, Gehr L, McDowell F: The dexamethasone suppression test: An indicator of depression in stroke but not a predictor of rehabilitation outcome. *Arch Neurol* 42:209-212, 1985

Schenkman M, Butler RB, Naeser MA, Kleefield J: Cerebral hemisphere asymmetry in CT and functional recovery from hemiplegia. *Neurology* 33:473-477, 1983

Smith DL, Akhtar AJ, Garraway WM: Proprioception and spatial neglect after stroke. *Age and Ageing* 12:63-69, 1983

Starr LB, Robinson RG, Price TR: Reliability, validity, and clinical utility of the social functioning exam in the assessment of stroke patients. *Experimental Aging Research* 9:101-106, 1983

Strand T, Asplund K, Eriksson S, Hagg E, Lithner F, Wester PO: A non-intensive stroke unit reduces functional disability and the need for long-term hospitalization. *Stroke* 16:29-34, 1985

Stroker R: Impact of disability on families of stroke clients. *J Neurosurgical Nurs* 15:360-365, 1983

Trombly CA, Quintana LA: Differences in responses to exercise by post-CVA and normal subjects. *Occup Ther J Research* 5:39-58, 1985

Wade DT, Hewer RL, Wood VA: Stroke: Influence of patient's sex and side of weakness on outcome. *Arch Phys Med Rehab* 65:513-516, 1984

Wade DT, Skilbeck CE, Hewer RL, Wood VA: Therapy after stroke: Amounts, determinants and effects. *Int Rehab Med* 6:105-110, 1984

Wade DT, Skilbeck CE, Wood VA, Hewer RL: Long-term survival after stroke. *Age and Ageing* 13:76-82, 1984

Wade DT, Wood VA, Hewer RL: Recovery after stroke--the first 3 months. *J Neurology, Neurosurgery, and Psychiatry* 48:7-13, 1985

Wilson DJ, Baker LL, Craddock JA: Functional test for the hemiparetic upper extremity. *Am J Occup Ther* 38:159-164, 1984

# PRINCIPAL CONTRIBUTORS

**Barbara E. Joe**, MA, is a quality assurance and program evaluation specialist in the Quality Assurance Division of the American Occupational Therapy Association. Her responsibilities include speaking, writing, and consulting on patient care evaluation.

**Kathy L. Kaplan**, MS, OTR, is a consultant to the American Occupational Therapy Association on the Efficacy Data Project. She is also a doctoral candidate in organizational behavior and development at George Washington University.

**Deborah Lieberman**, MA, OTR, is the director of occupational therapy at the National Rehabilitation Hospital in Washington, D.C. Her specialty areas are physical disabilities and administration.

**Susan C. Merrill**, MA, OTR, is an instructor in the Department of Occupational Therapy at Thomas Jefferson University in Philadelphia. Pediatrics, juvenile arthritis, and research methodology are her teaching fields.

**Patricia C. Ostrow**, MA, OTR, FAOTA, is the director of the American Occupational Therapy Association's Quality Assurance Division. She conceptualized the Efficacy Data Project and brought it to fruition.

**Kenneth J. Ottenbacher**, PhD, OTR, FAOTA, is an assistant professsor in the School of Allied Health Professions, University of Wisconsin-Madison. He teaches research methods to undergraduate students and pediatric developmental disabilities to graduate students.

# INDEX OF AUTHORS OF ABSTRACTED ARTICLES

Wolcott LE    76
Wolf SL    77
Yu J    78
Zuger RR    75
Zutshi DW    63

The American Occupational Therapy Association is interested in the outcomes of this book on stroke outcomes. Please answer the following questions so that future books can be tailored to the needs of members.

1. How useful was this book to you? Rate the usefulness on a scale of 1 to 10, 1 being totally useless and 10 being extremely useful.___
   Explain how the book was useful._____
   _____
   _____
   Explain how you would increase the usefulness of the book.
   _____
   _____

2. Would you like to see the book expanded? Yes ___ No ___
   If yes, in which areas?_____

3. Would you like to see books like this on topics other than stroke? Yes ___ No ____
   If yes, on what topics? _____

4. Are you a clinician ___, researcher ___, teacher ___, student ___, manager ___, or other ___?

5. Check below the Efficacy Data Briefs that you would like to receive, free of charge.
   _____ *Research Shows Shorter Hospitalization Related to Occupational Therapy.* March 1983
   _____ *Outpatient Stroke Therapy Reduces Functional Deterioration.* March 1983
   _____ *Stroke Rehabilitation, Including Occupational Therapy as Part of Team, Shows Statistically Significant Long-Term Functional Gains.* March 1983

MAIL YOUR COMPLETED SURVEY AND ORDER FORM TO

American Occupational Therapy Association
1383 Piccard Drive
Rockville, MD 20850